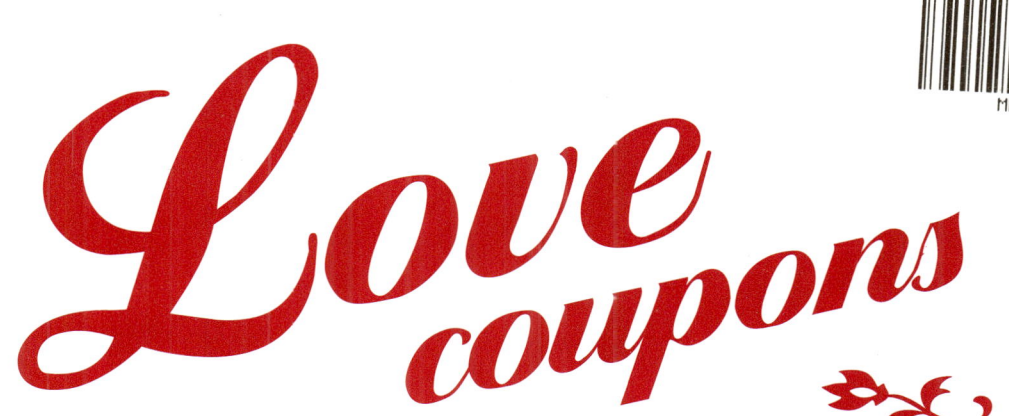

Love coupons

Don Byrd and Leanna Wolfe

Published by LONGSTREET PRESS, INC.,
a subsidiary of Cox Newspapers, a division of Cox Enterprises, Inc.
2140 Newmarket Parkway, Suite 118
Marietta, Georgia 30067

Printed in the United States of America

1st printing, 1994

ISBN: 1-56352-178-4

This book was printed by Vaughan Printing, Nashville, Tennessee

Book and cover design by Jill Dible

Love Coupons ❧ A User's Guide

Note to Buyers:

When you buy these for a lover, you may want to remove the ones that aren't really appropriate for your relationship (e.g., No Kids Weekend, Kinky Sex Adventure, Designated Drinker), but don't pull out too many. These coupons can be your opportunity to indulge each other — to sleep in late, to go away for the weekend, or to explore an erotic fantasy. Don't forget to invent some of your own by using the blank forms in the back.

When you give *Love Coupons*, you give that special person in your life permission to be difficult, but still be loved. Instead of resenting your lover for fighting, complaining or being critical, just redeem his or her coupon for Immediate End To An Argument or Two Hours To Whine And Complain. Then, rather than resisting the opportunity to be close, you can both focus on enjoying each other.

Note to Receivers:

Welcome to the world of *Love Coupons*. As the receiver of this very special gift, you must know that someone loves you. What's more, someone loves you just as you are; and to prove it, you're being offered — among other things — permission not to make sense, to drink to your heart's content at the next party, and to indulge in a no-questions night out.

Of course, your lover also wants to pamper you. You're now free to enjoy a Candlelight Dinner, a Total Chocolate Day, a Full Body Massage, a Total Indulgence Day, and to wallow in a Sensuous Bubble Bath. Your special person also wants to show you the many ways of love by offering you some Very Erotic Kisses, your very own Erotic Fantasy, a Night Of Love Slavery, and a Mystery Weekend designed just for you. Enjoy.

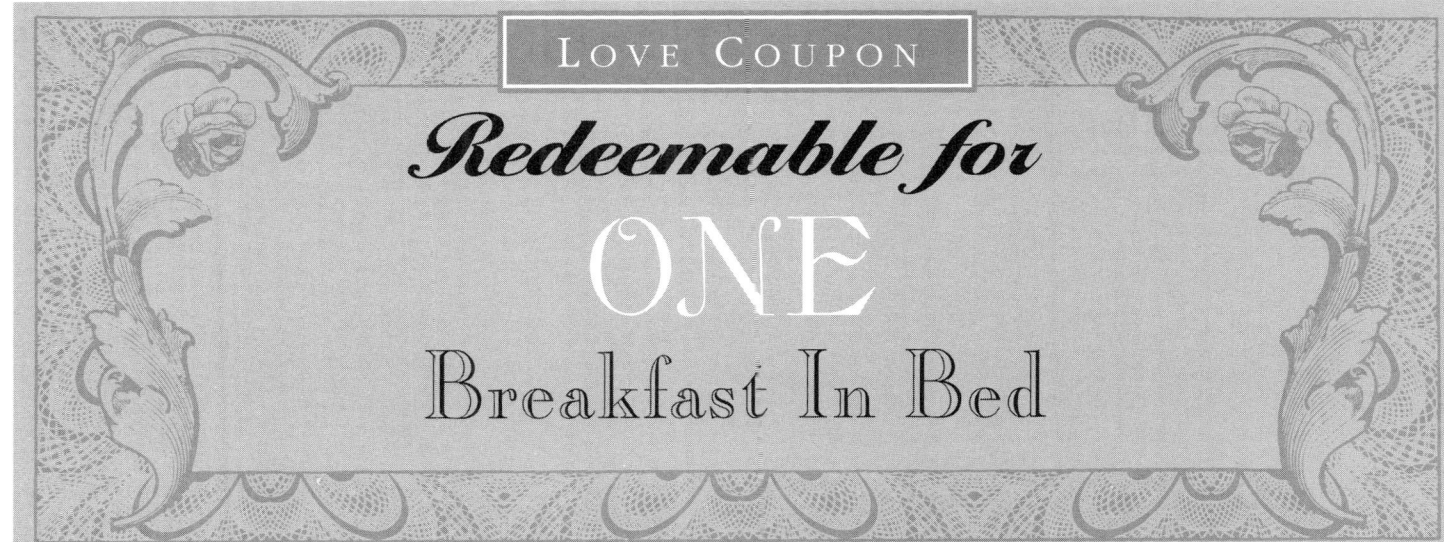

LOVE COUPON

Redeemable for

ONE

Breakfast In Bed

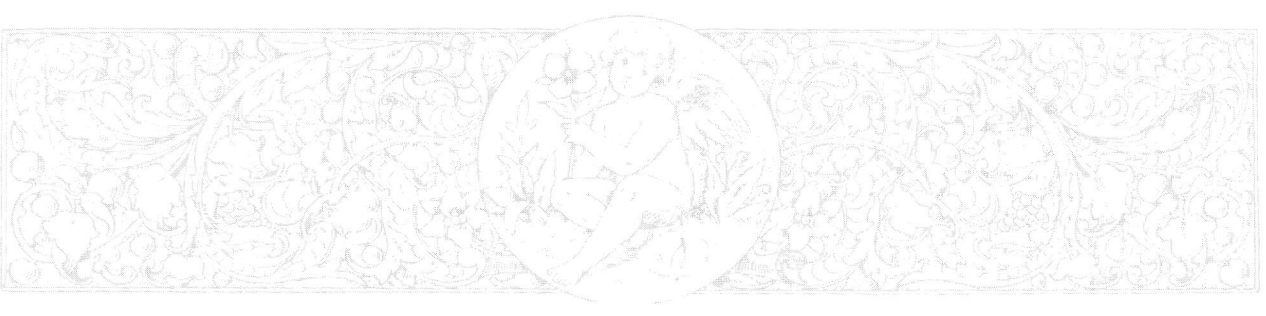

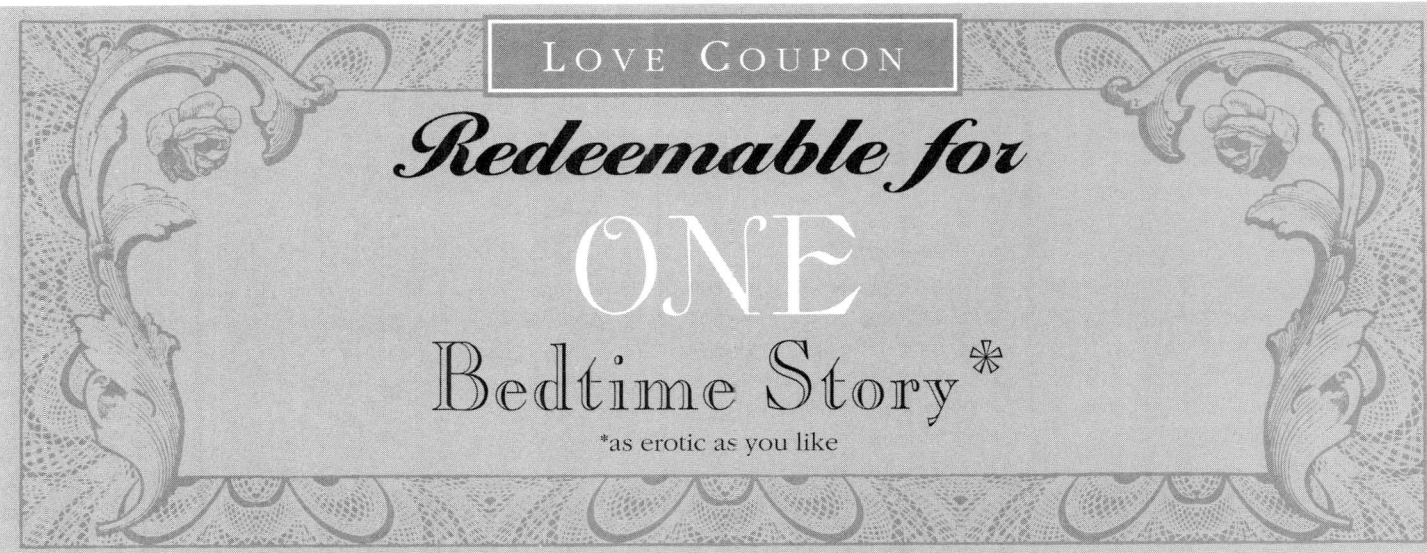

LOVE COUPON

Redeemable for

ONE

Bedtime Story*

*as erotic as you like

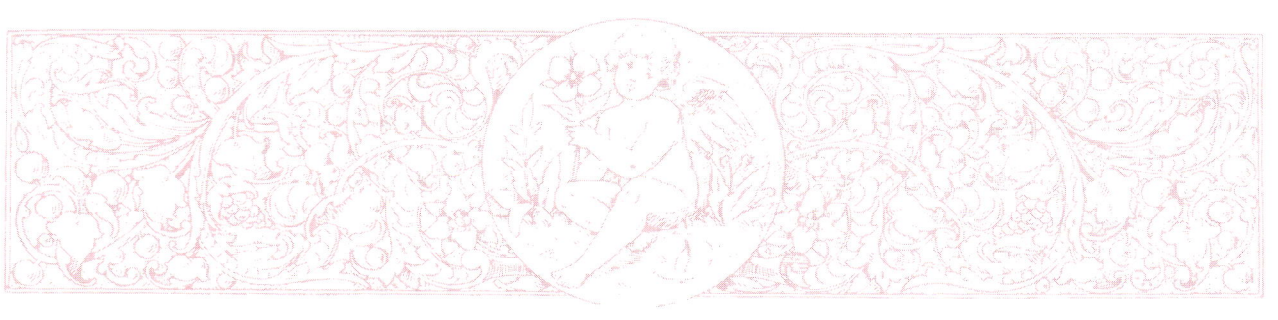

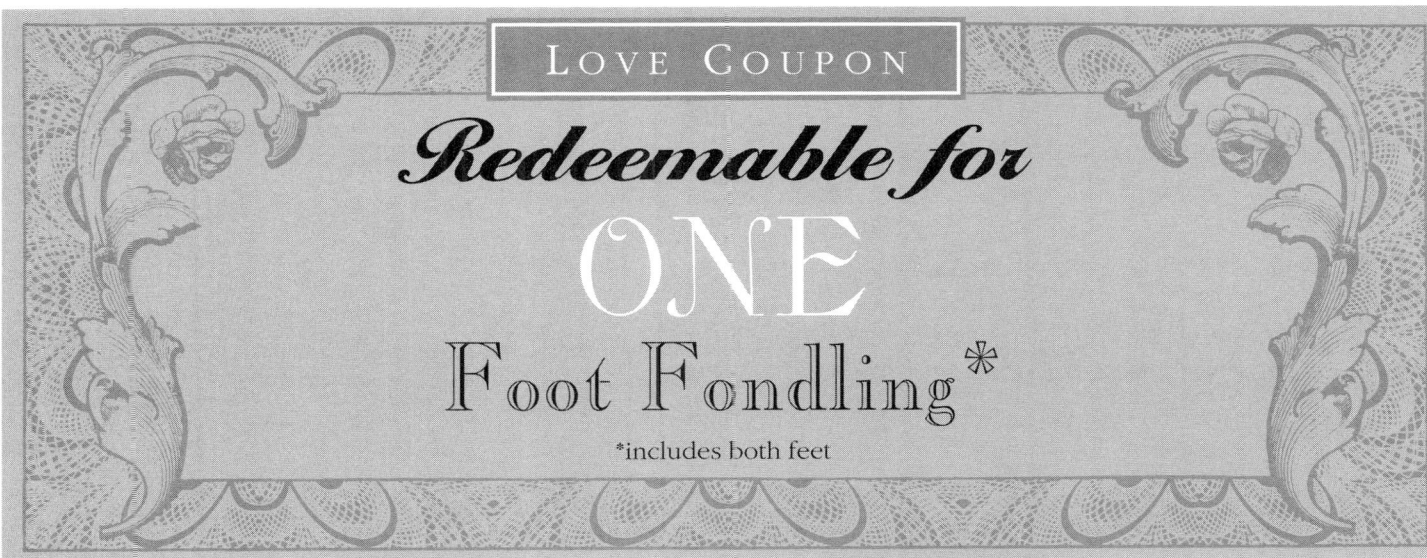

LOVE COUPON

Redeemable for

ONE

Foot Fondling*

*includes both feet

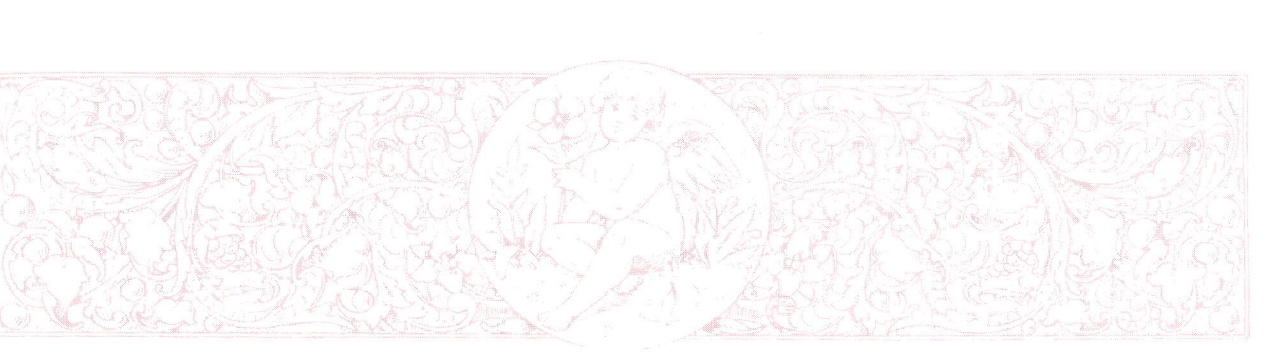

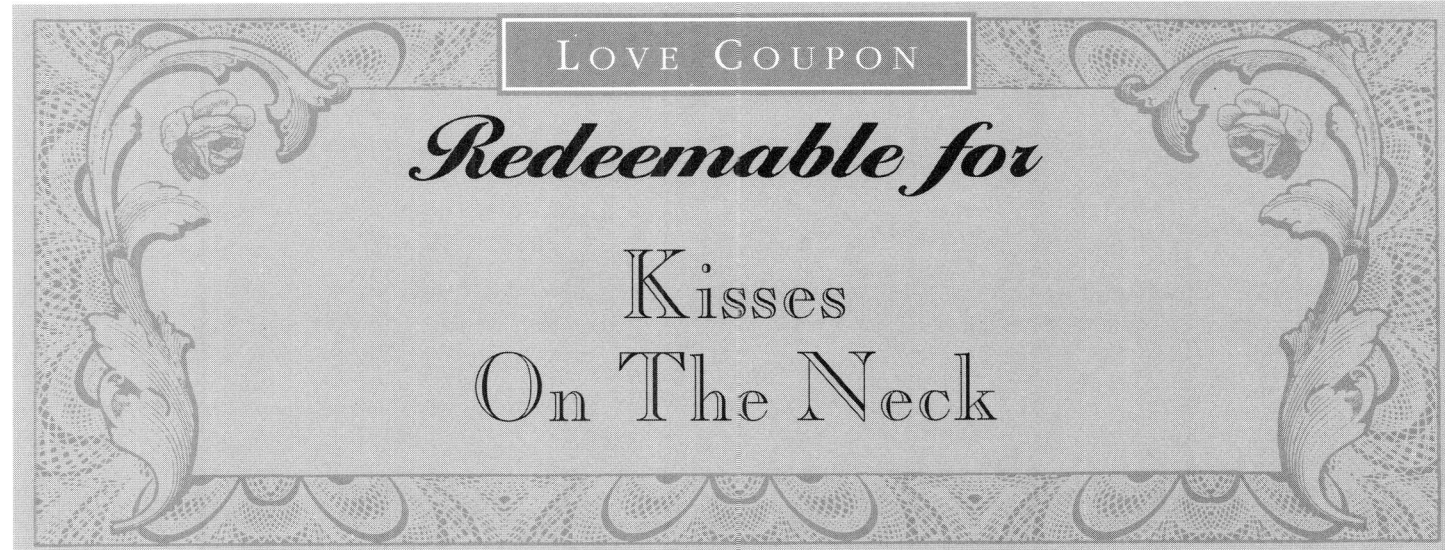

LOVE COUPON

Redeemable for

Kisses
On The Neck

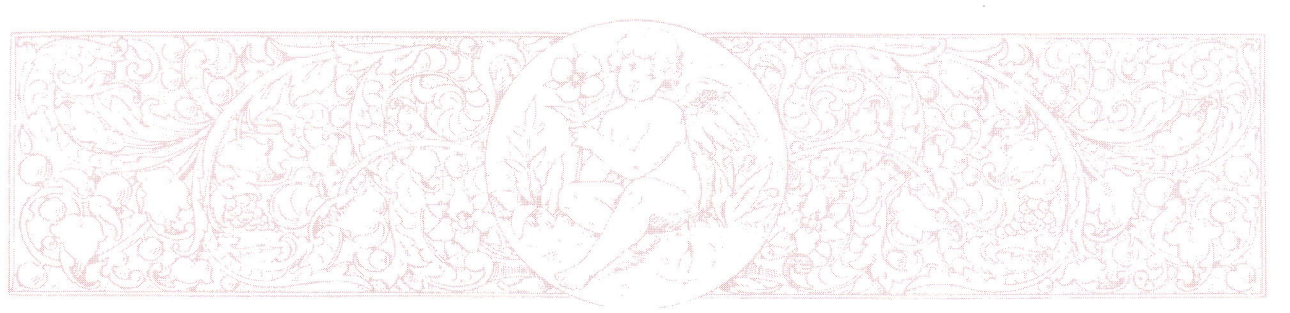

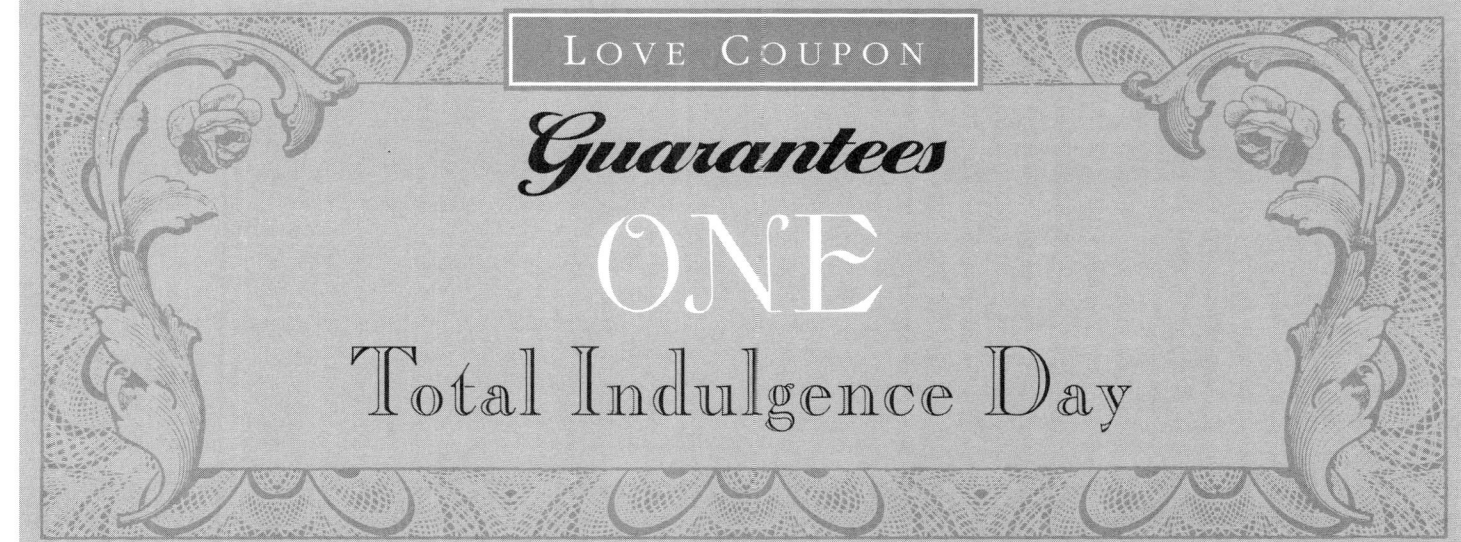

LOVE COUPON

Guarantees

ONE

Total Indulgence Day

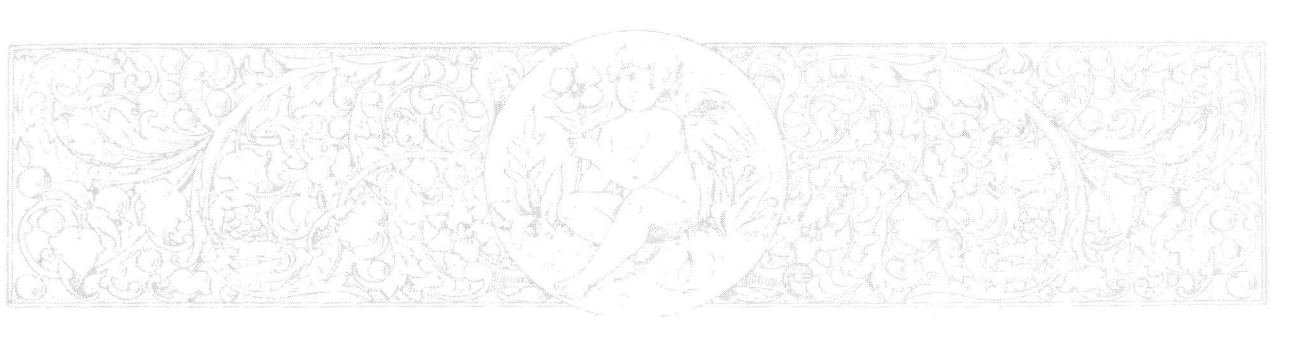

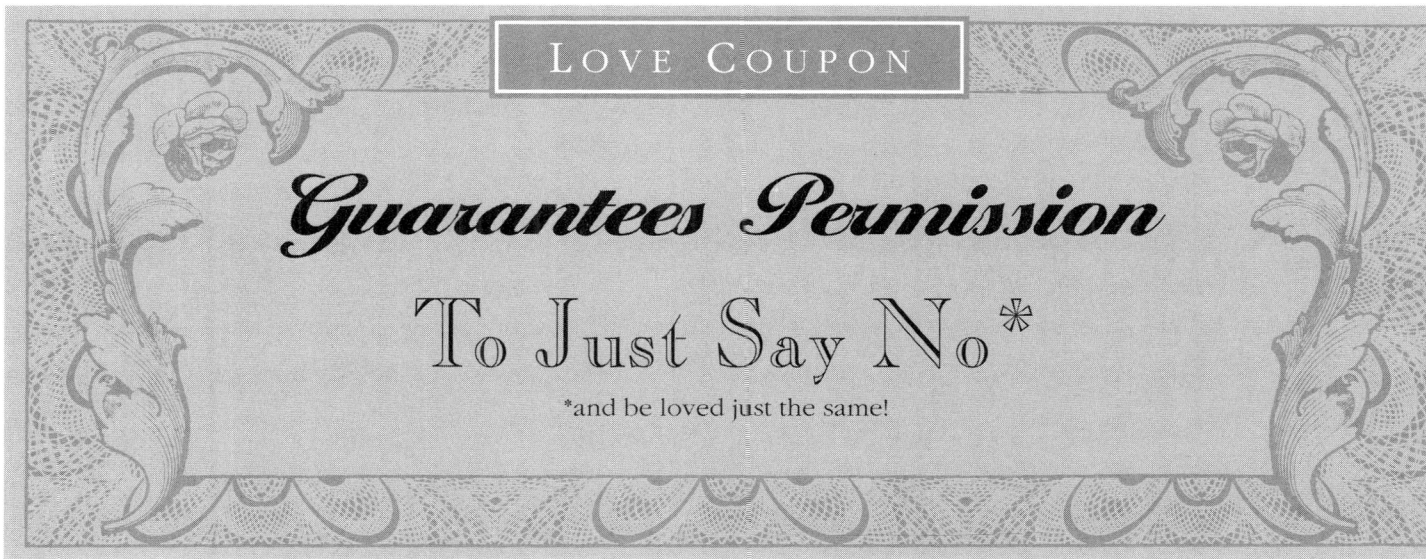

LOVE COUPON

Guarantees Permission

To Just Say No*

*and be loved just the same!

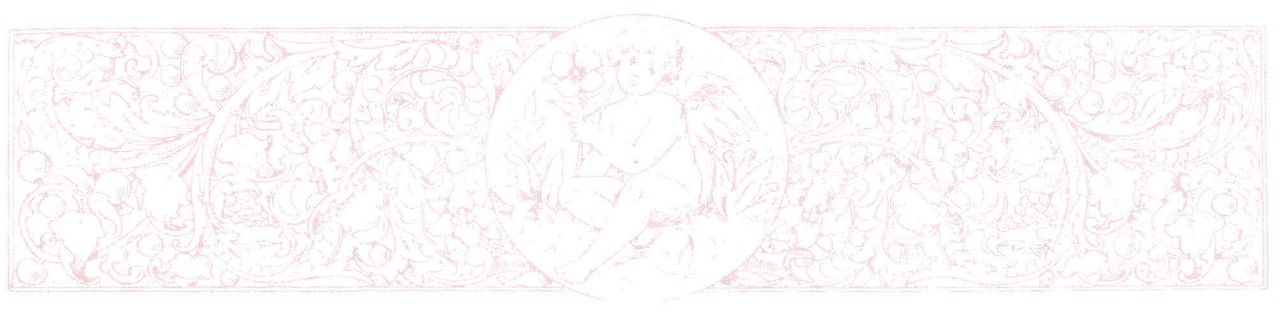

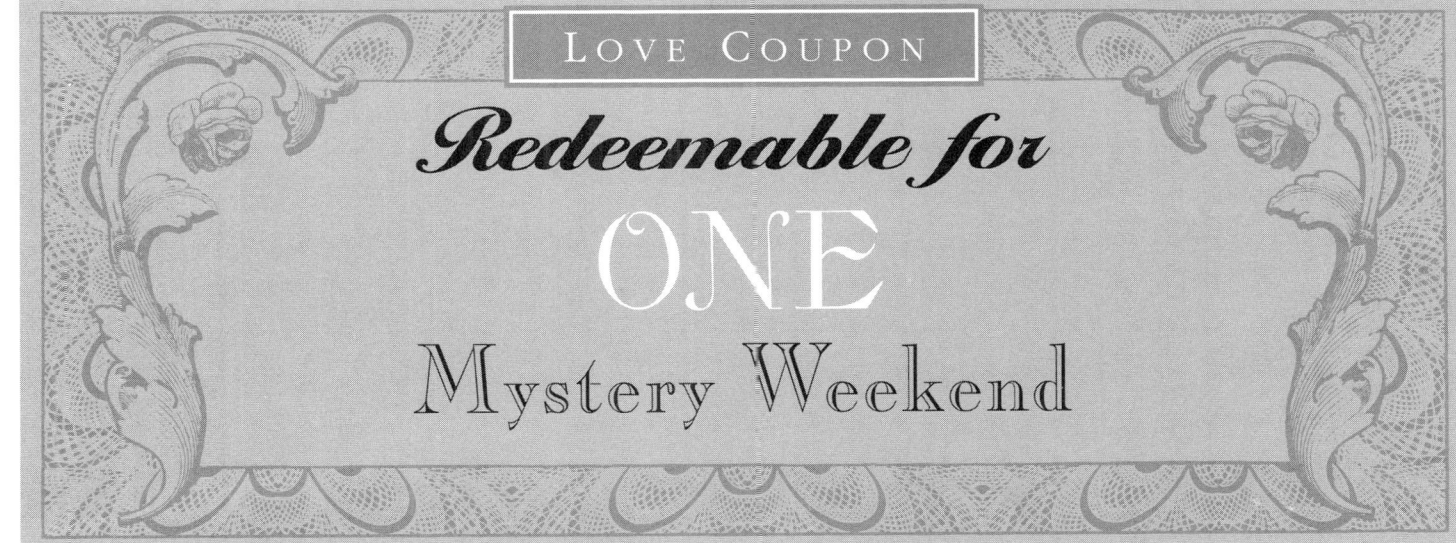

LOVE COUPON

Redeemable for

ONE

Mystery Weekend

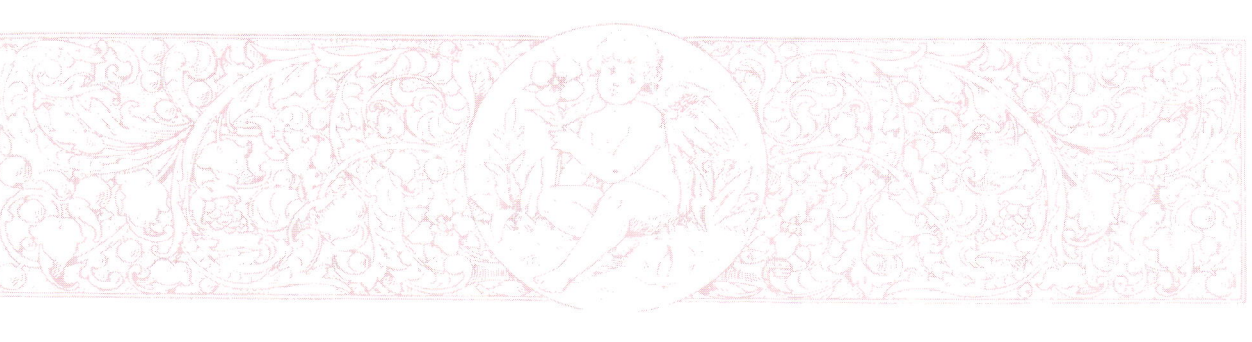

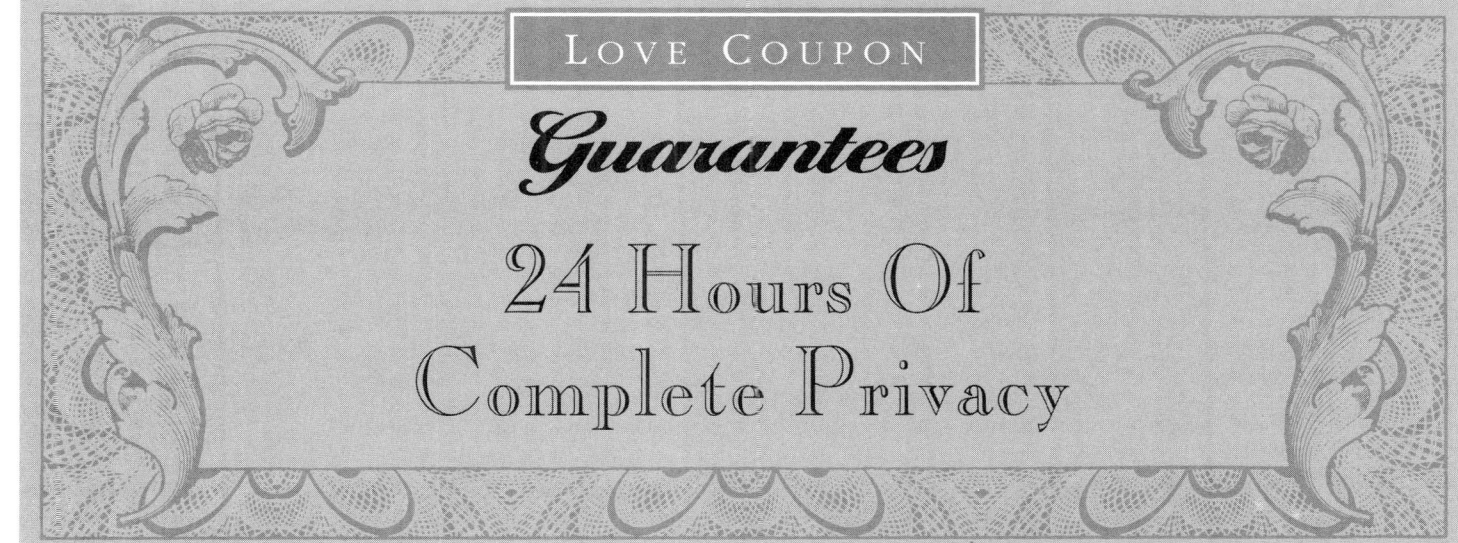

LOVE COUPON

Guarantees

24 Hours Of
Complete Privacy

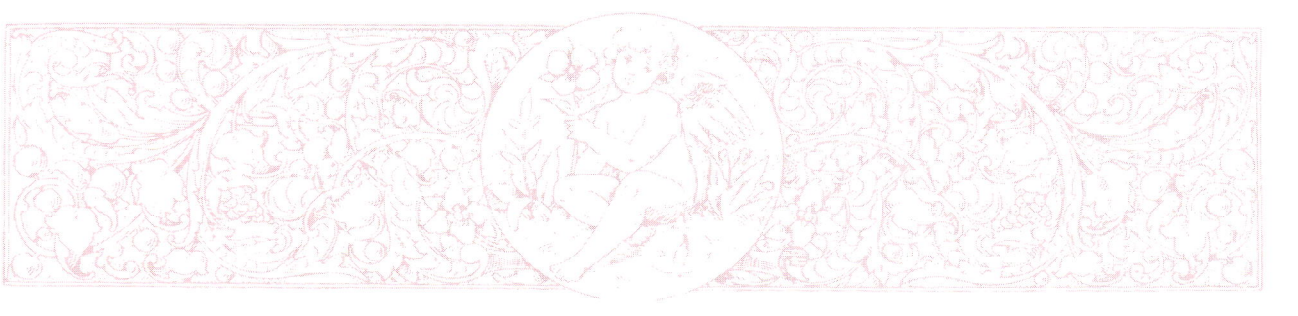

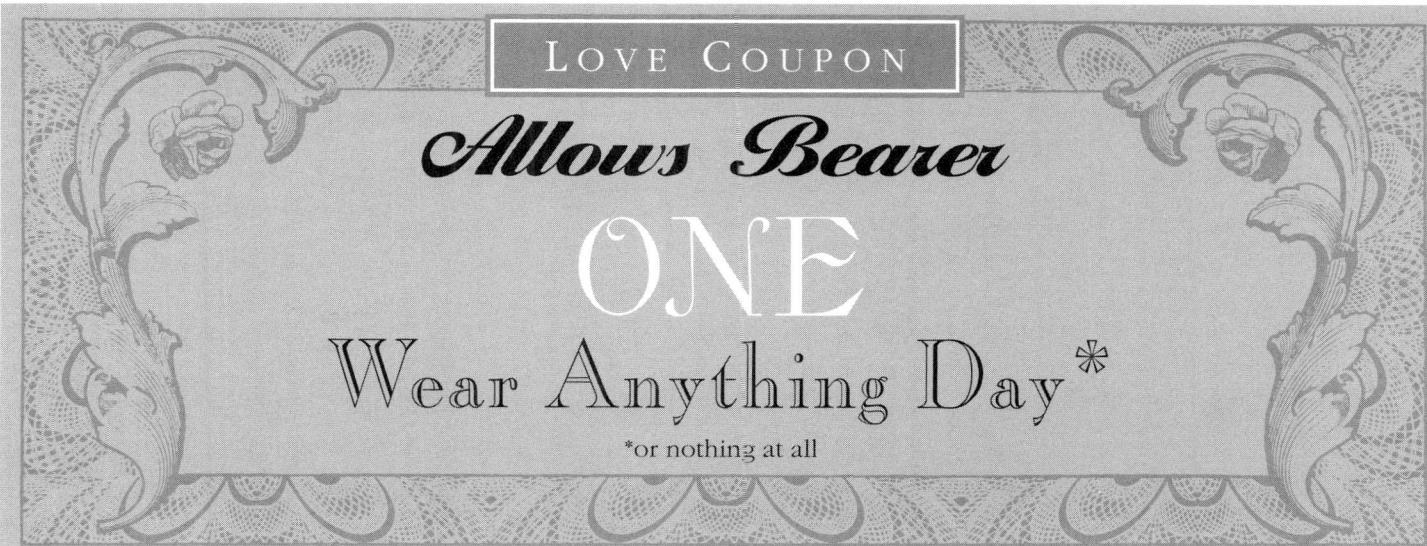

LOVE COUPON

Allows Bearer

ONE

Wear Anything Day*

*or nothing at all

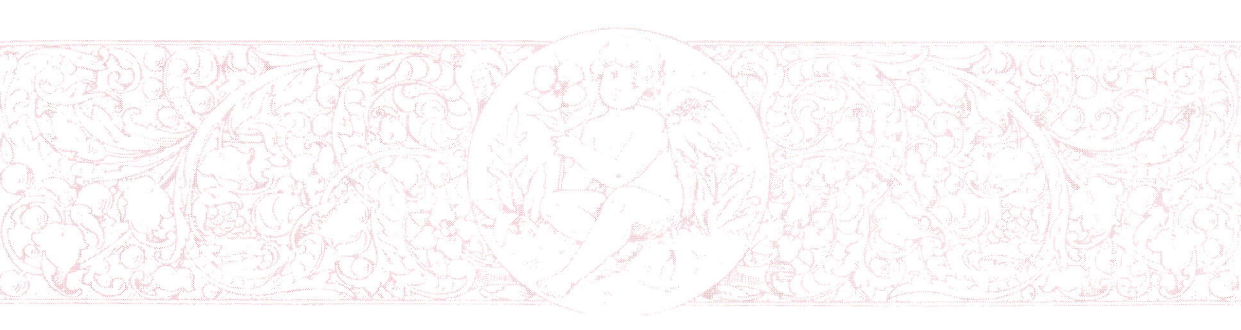

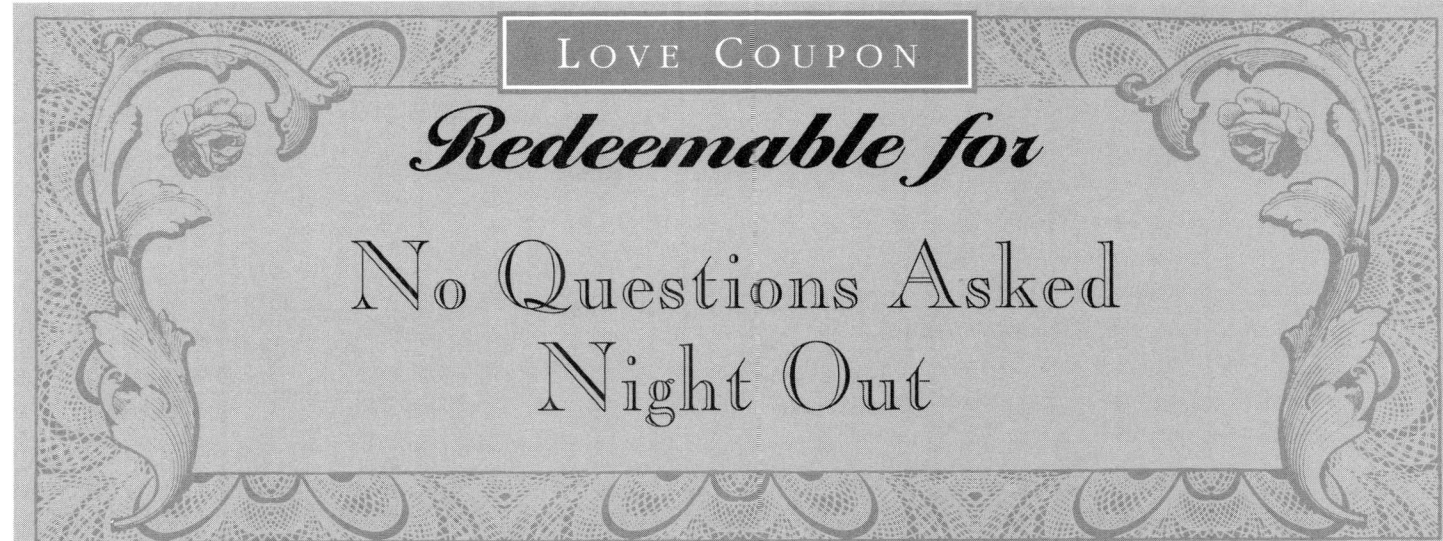

LOVE COUPON

Redeemable for

No Questions Asked
Night Out

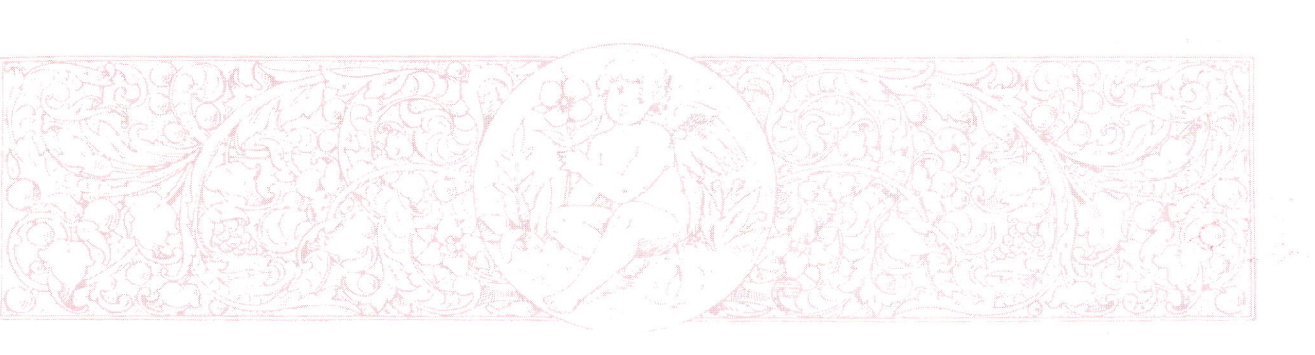

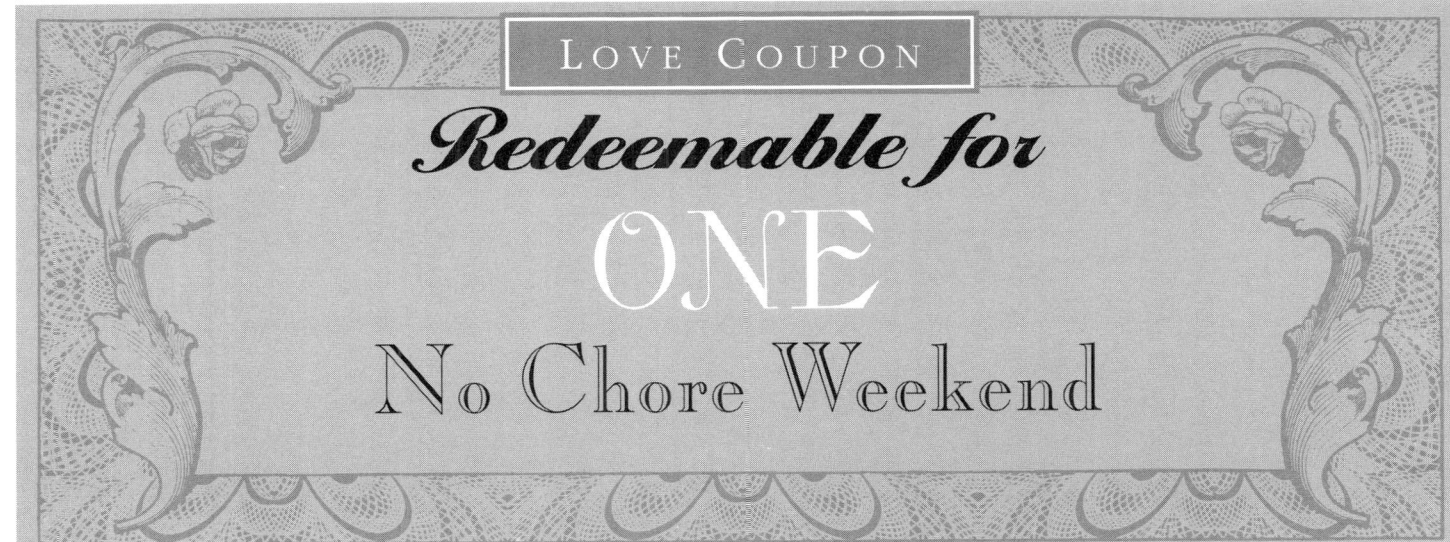

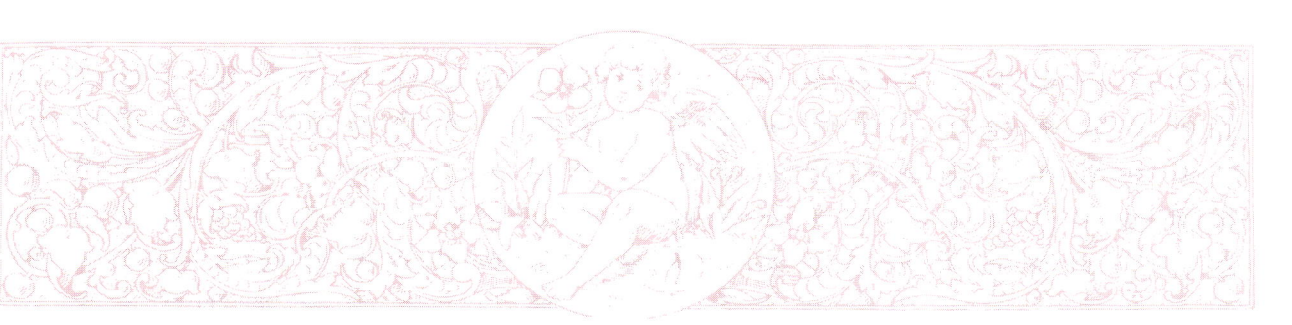

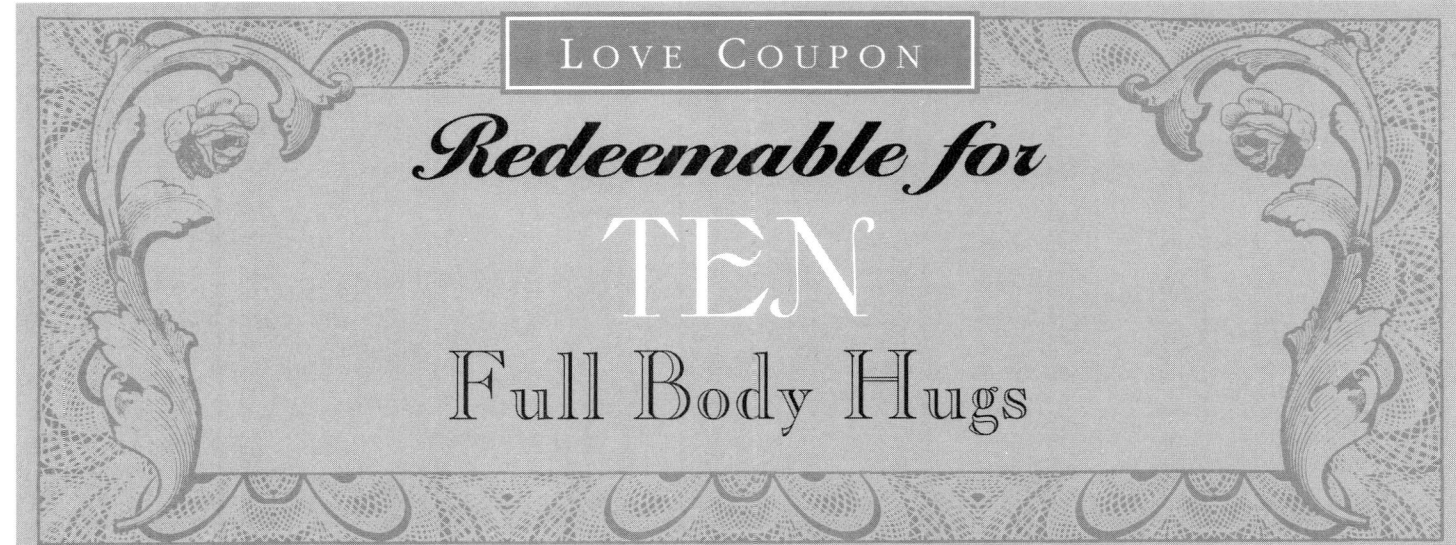

LOVE COUPON

Redeemable for

TEN

Full Body Hugs

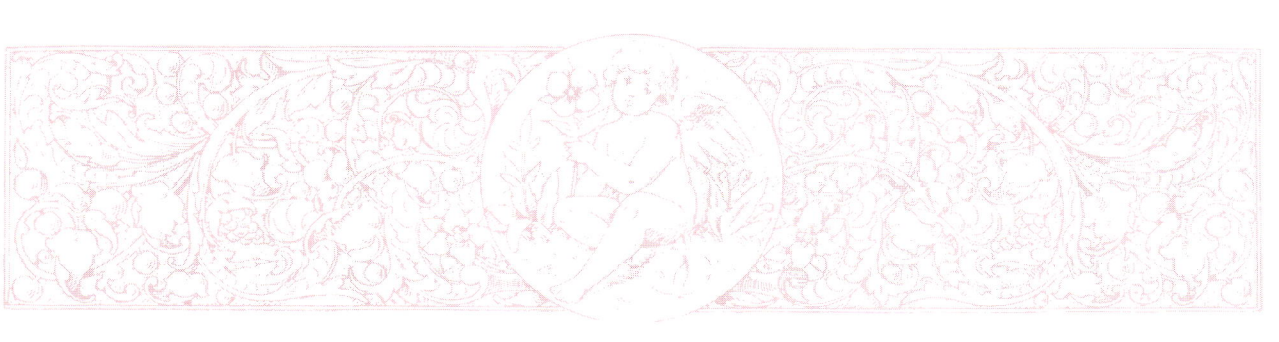

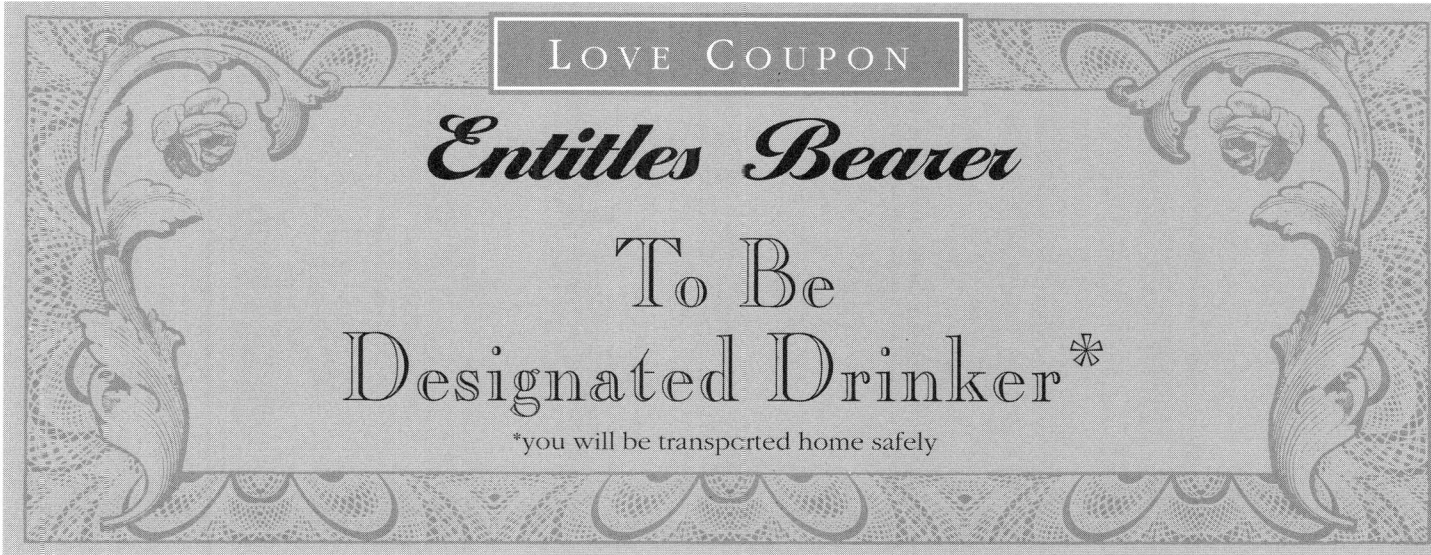

LOVE COUPON

Entitles Bearer

To Be

Designated Drinker*

*you will be transported home safely

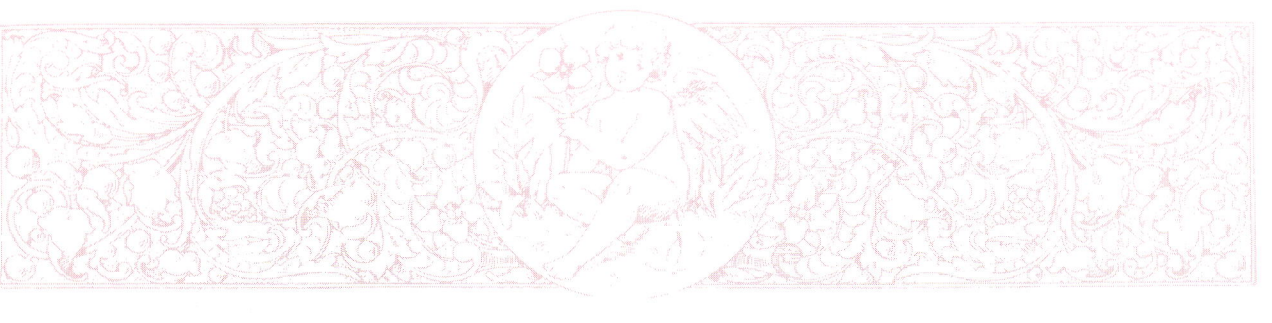

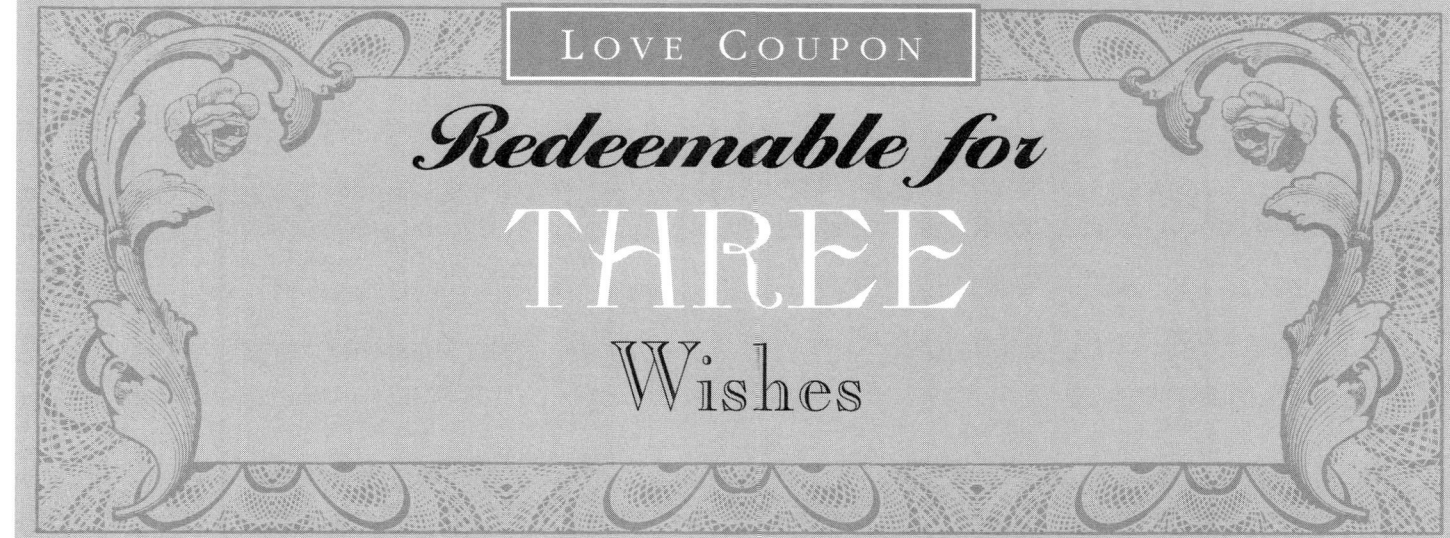

LOVE COUPON

Redeemable for

THREE

Wishes

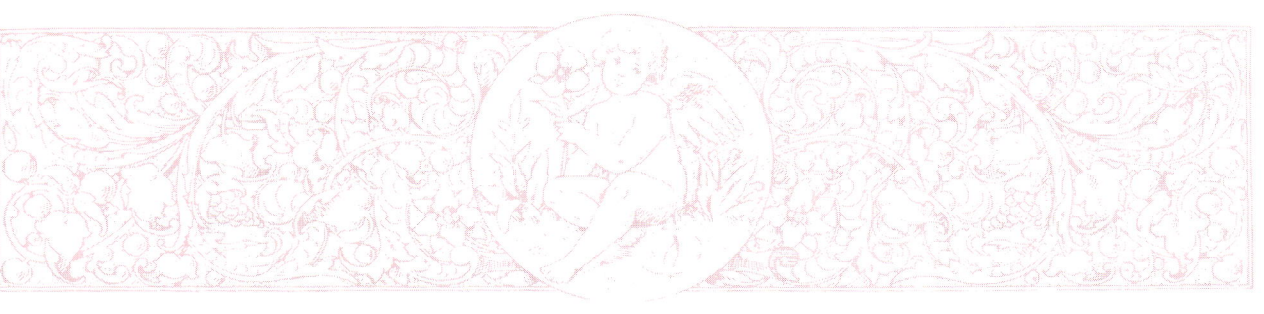

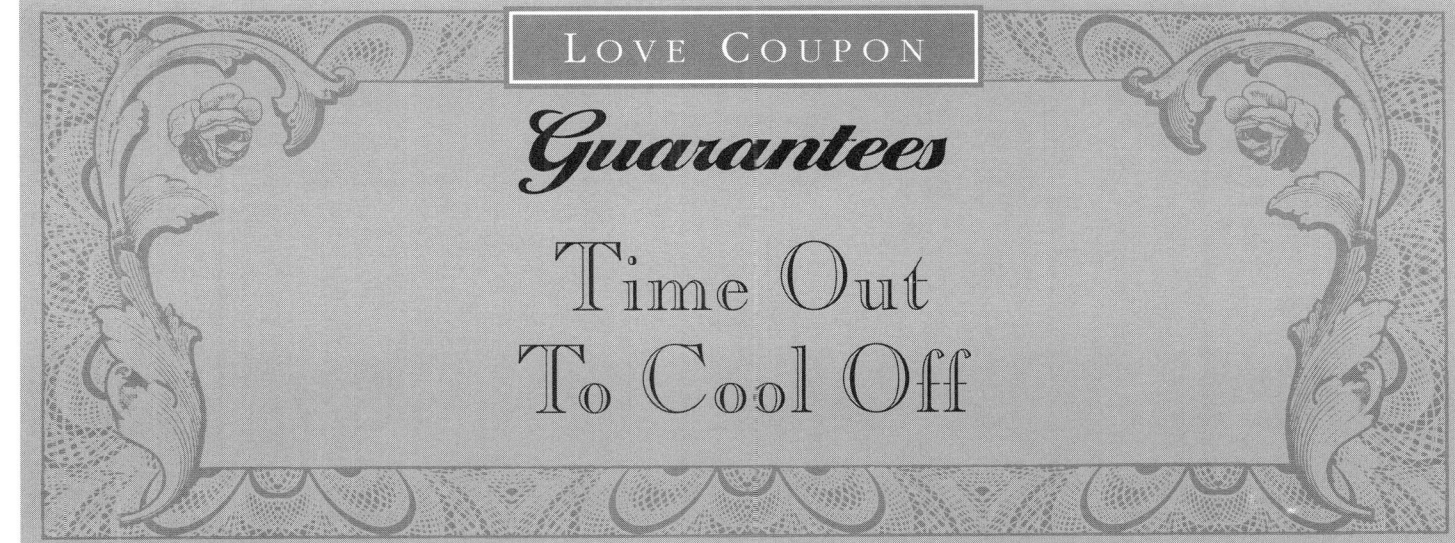

LOVE COUPON

Guarantees

Time Out
To Cool Off

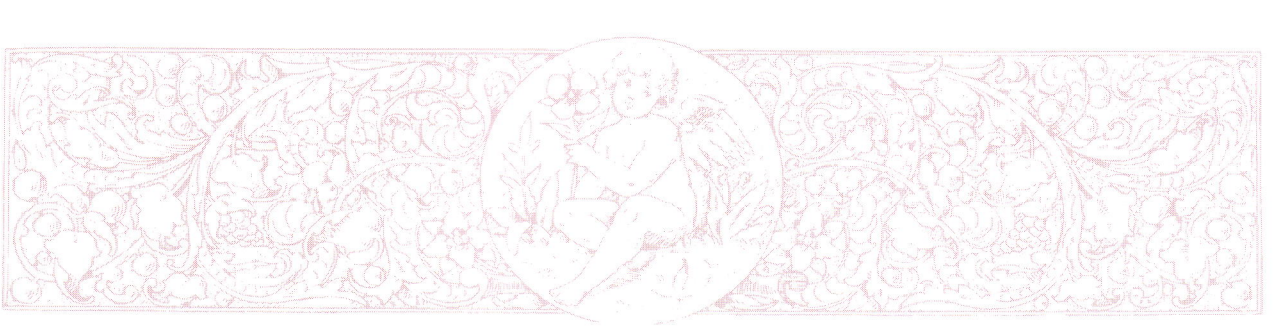

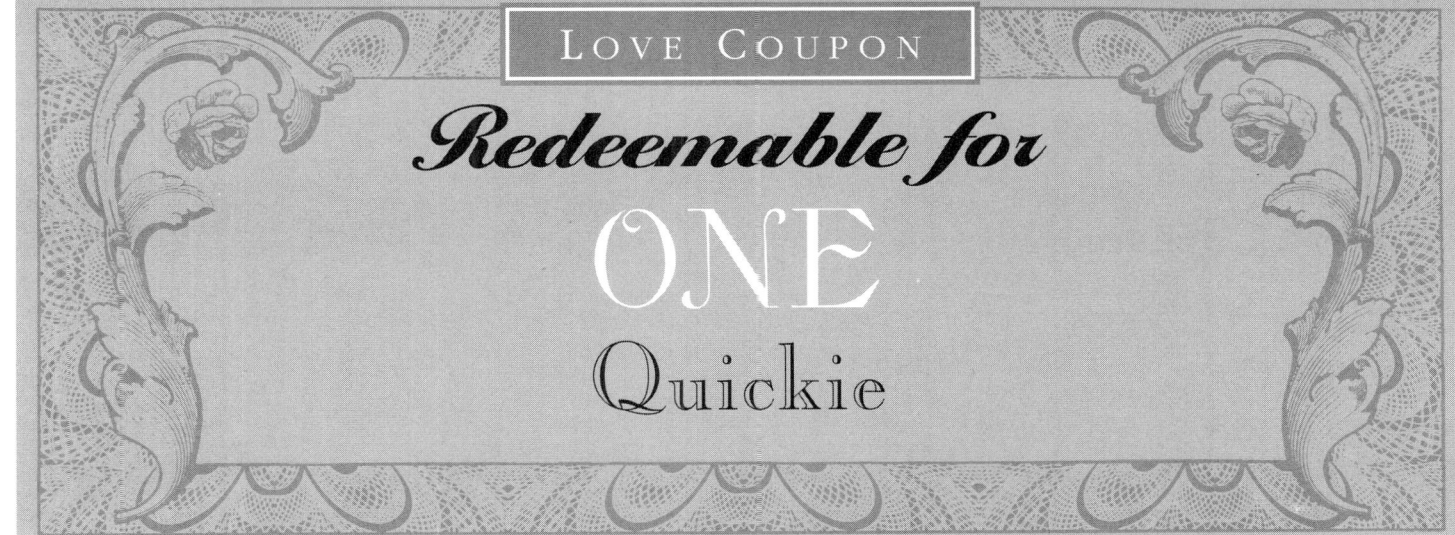

LOVE COUPON

Redeemable for

ONE

Quickie

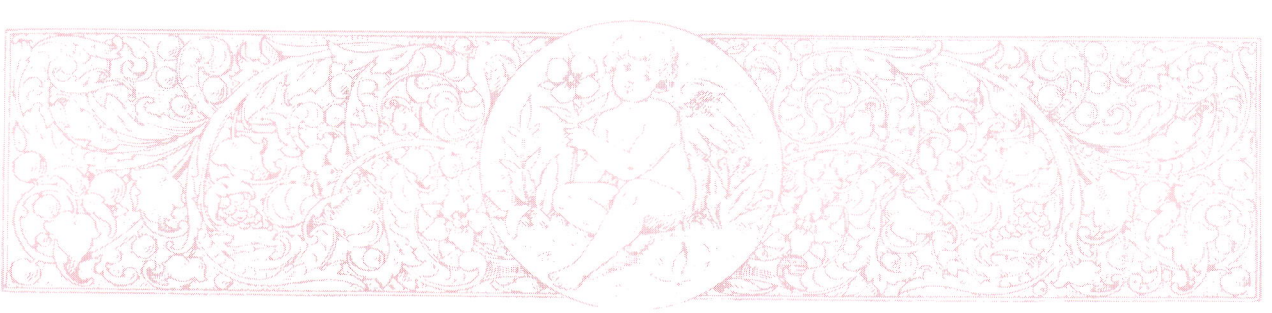

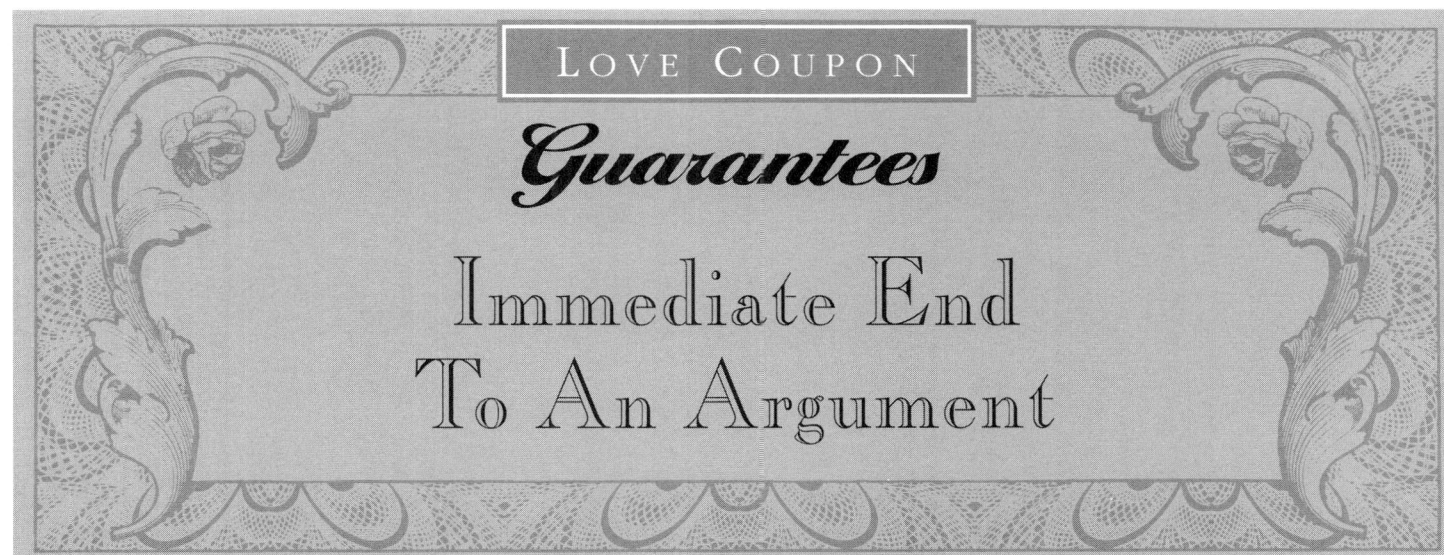

LOVE COUPON

Guarantees

Immediate End
To An Argument

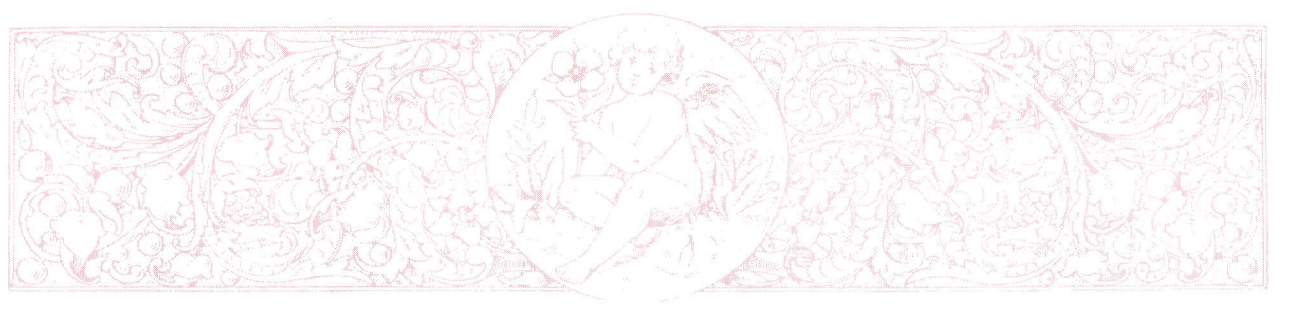

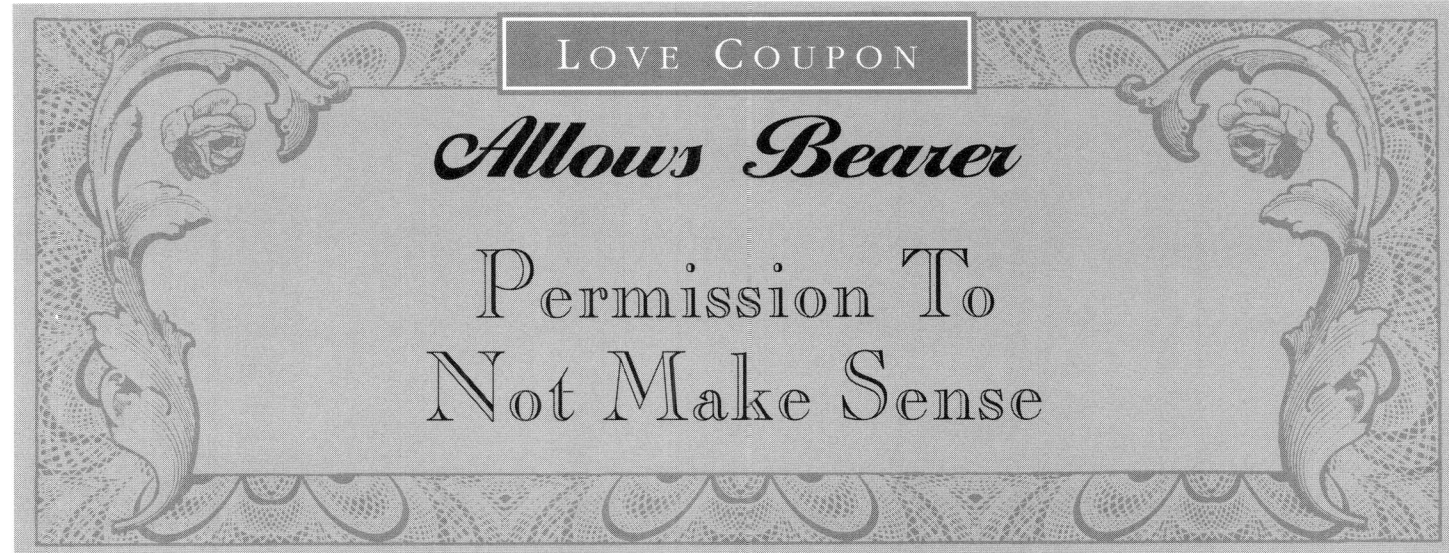

LOVE COUPON

Allows Bearer

Permission To
Not Make Sense

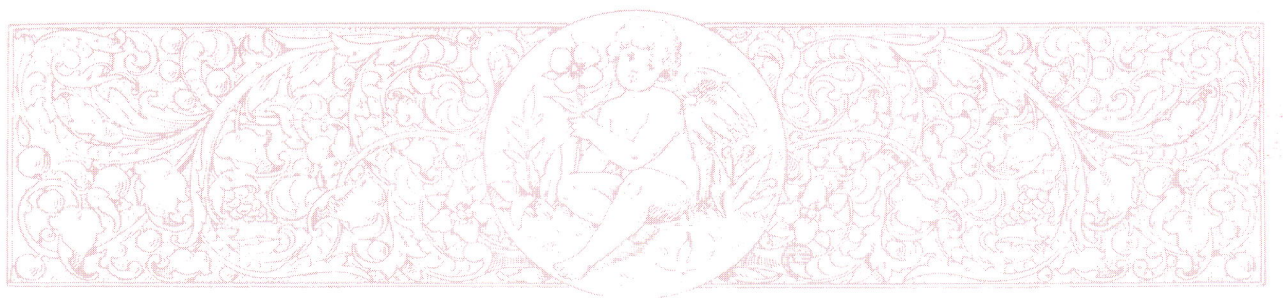

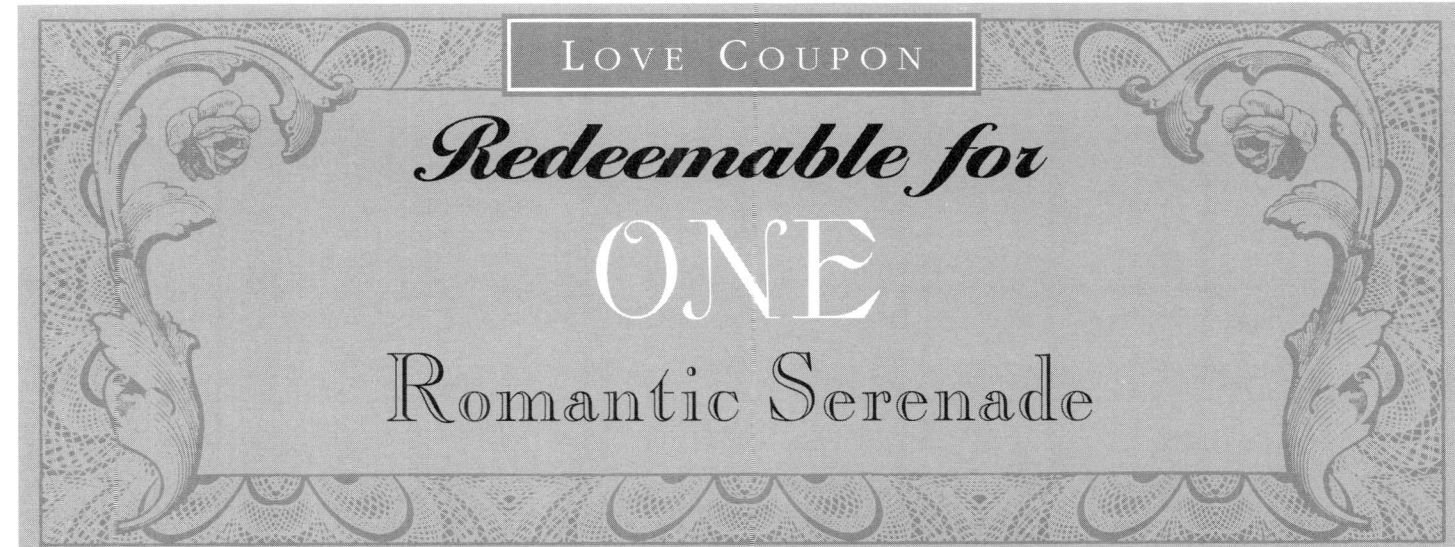

LOVE COUPON

Redeemable for

ONE

Romantic Serenade

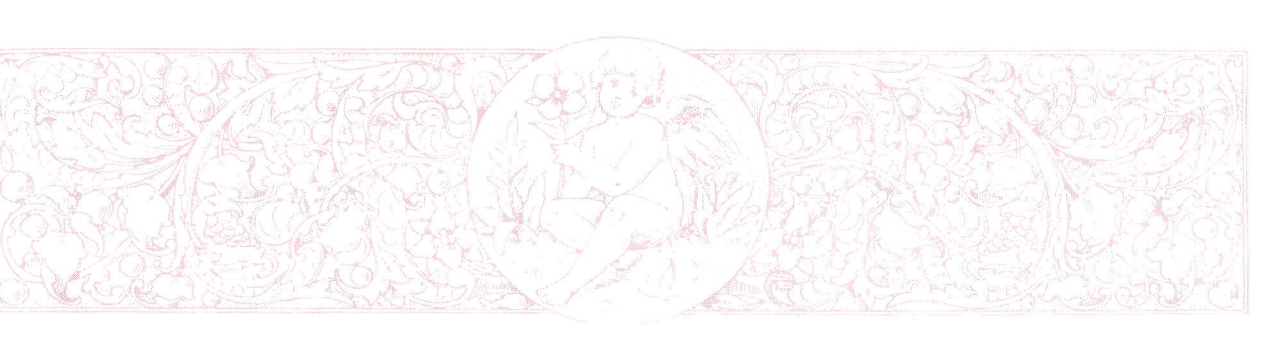

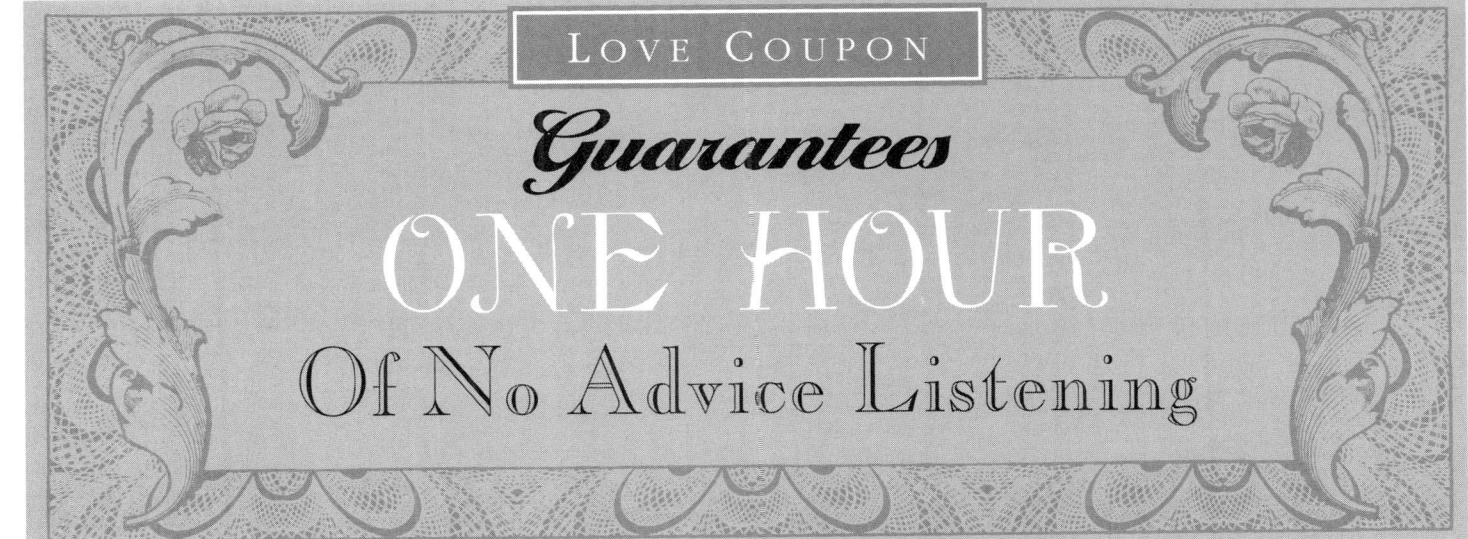

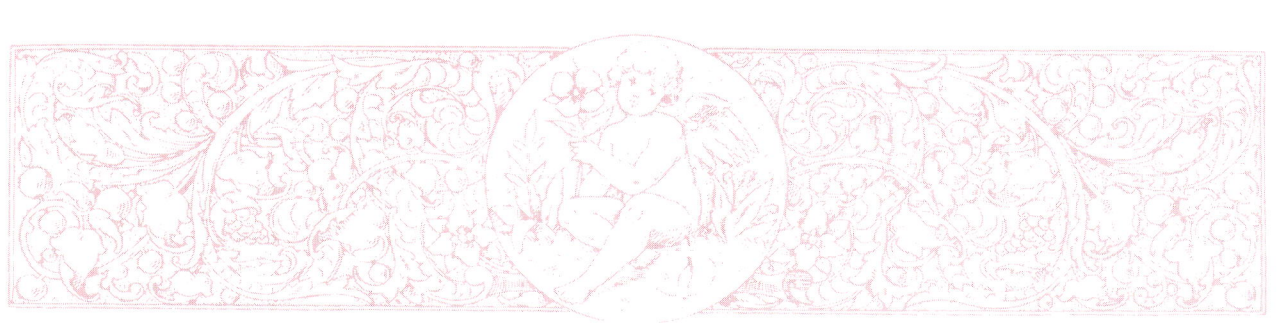

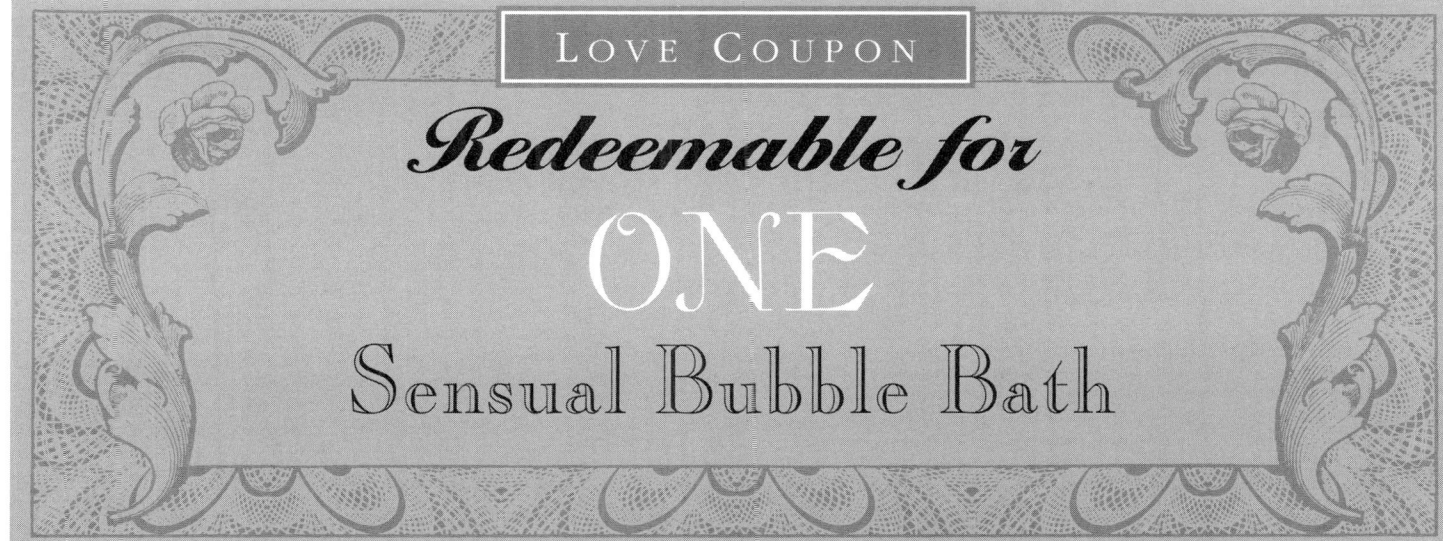

LOVE COUPON

Redeemable for

ONE

Sensual Bubble Bath

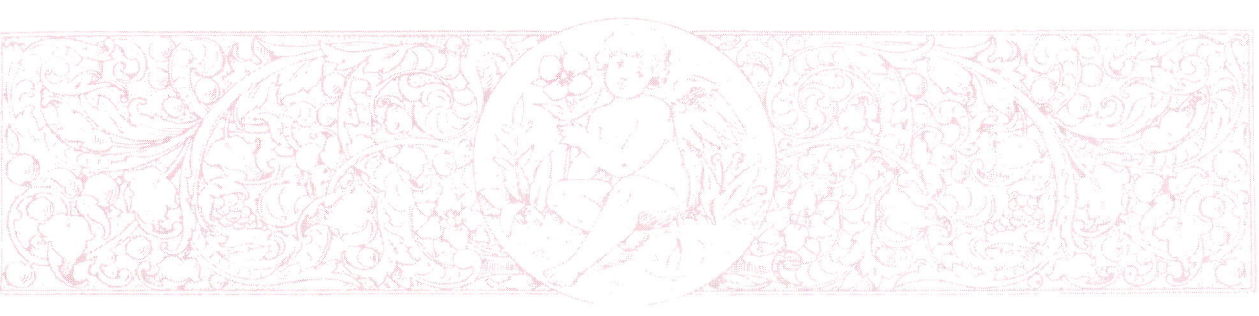

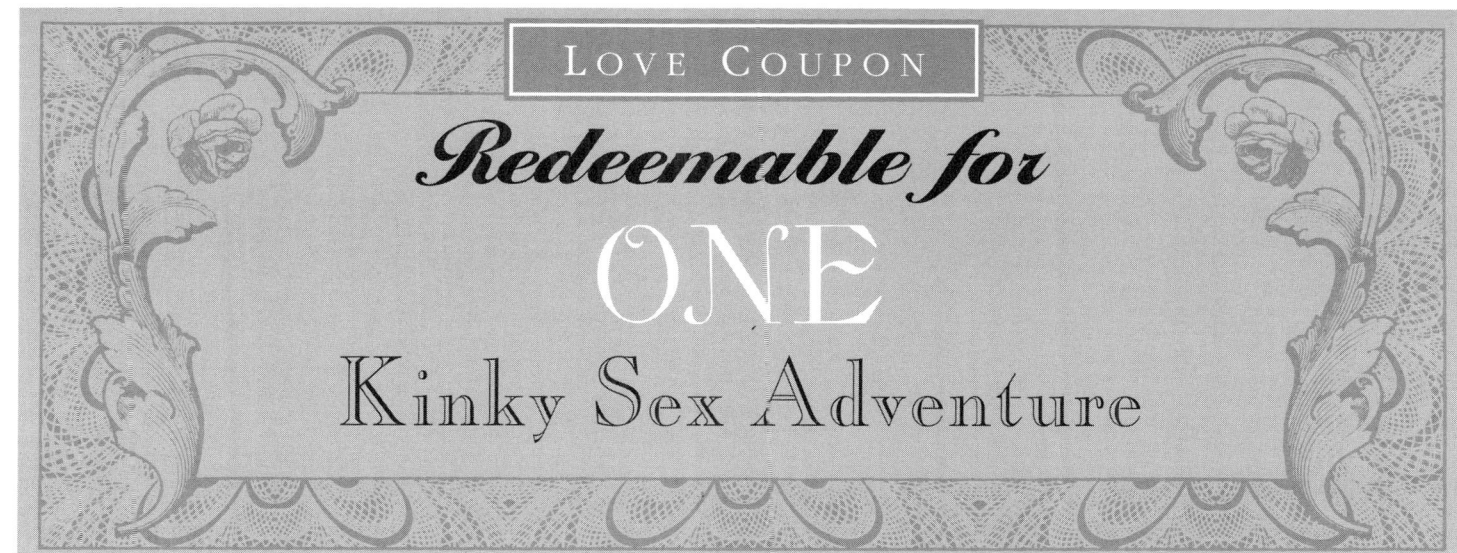

LOVE COUPON

Redeemable for

ONE

Kinky Sex Adventure

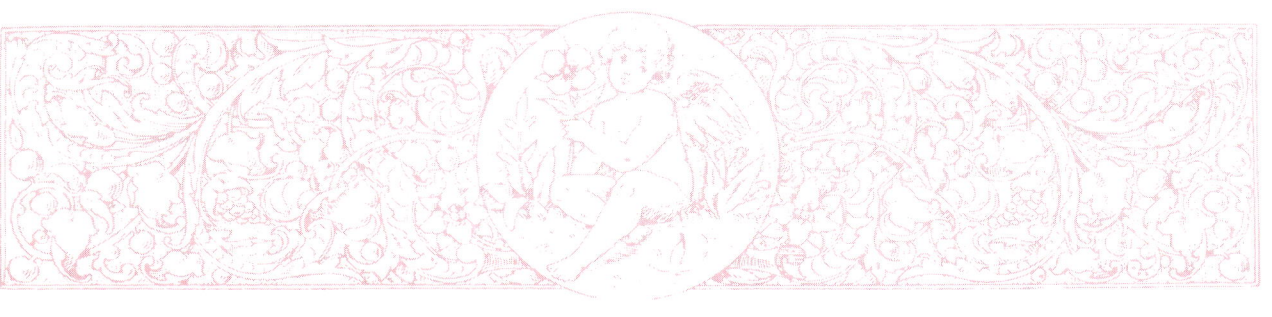

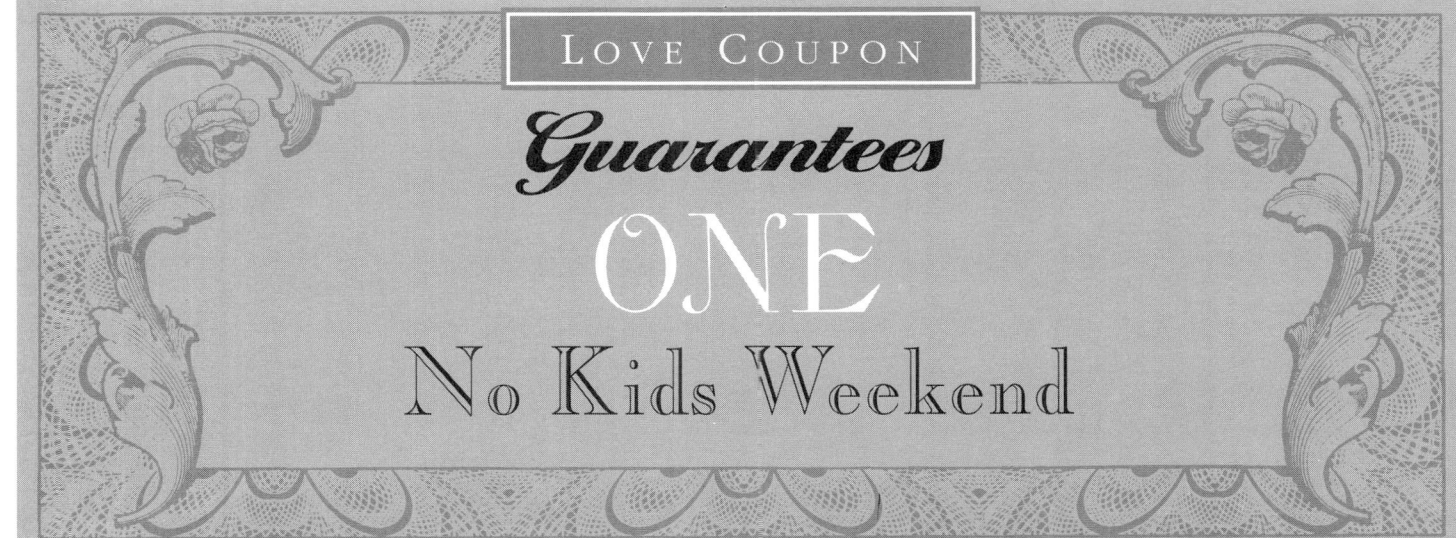

LOVE COUPON

Guarantees

ONE

No Kids Weekend

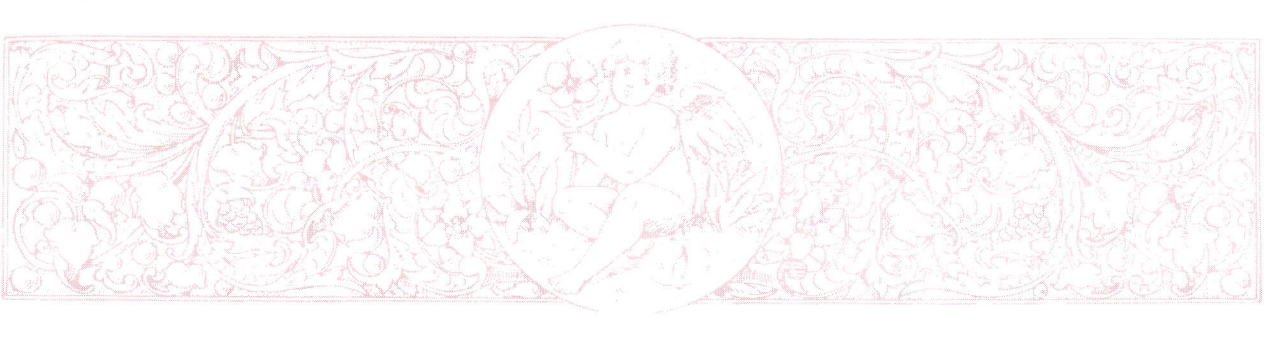

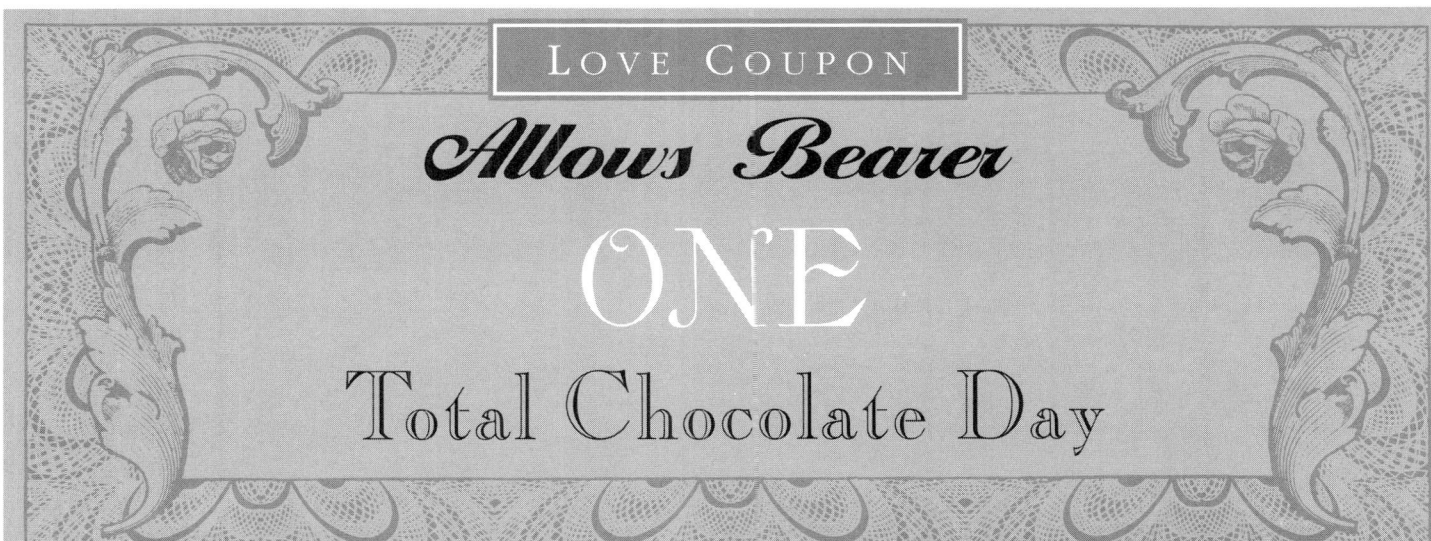

LOVE COUPON

Allows Bearer

ONE

Total Chocolate Day

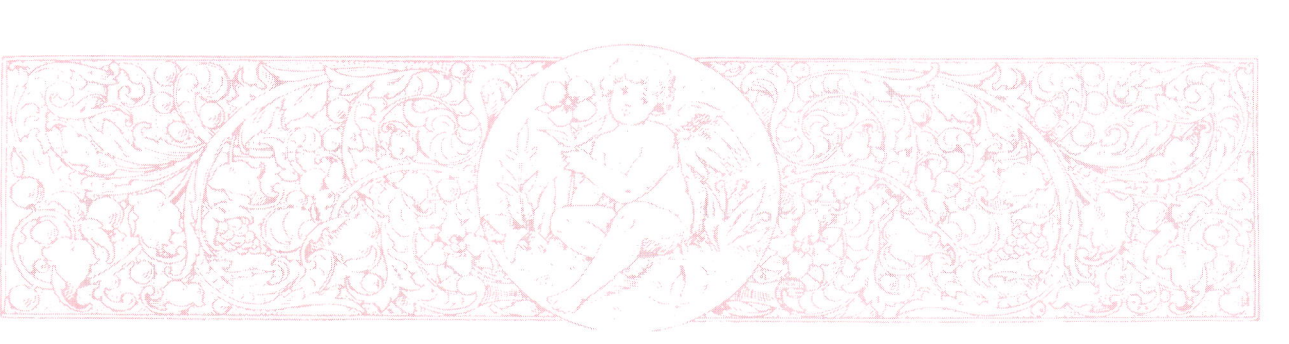

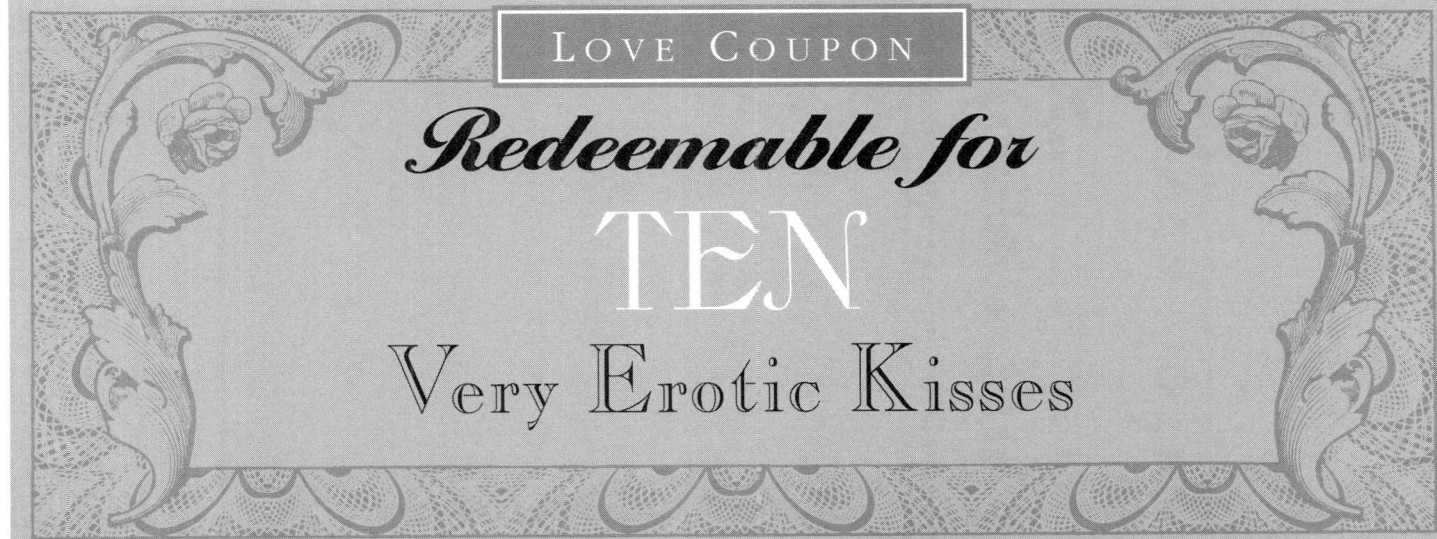

LOVE COUPON

Redeemable for

TEN

Very Erotic Kisses

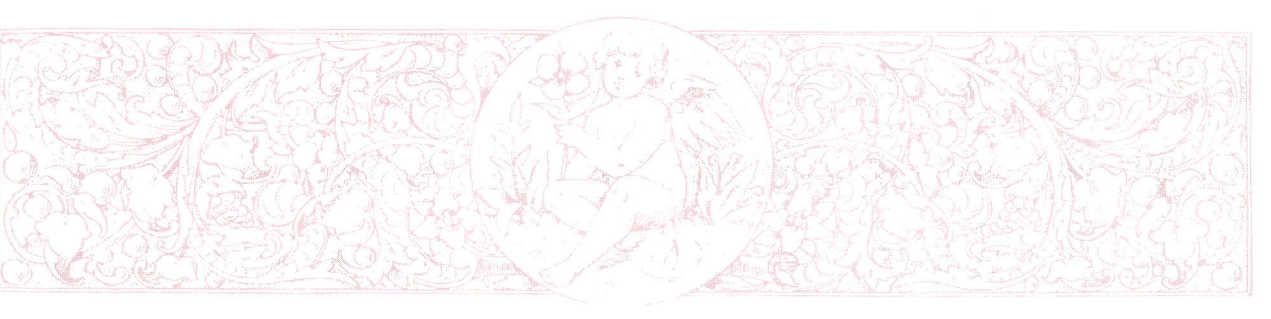

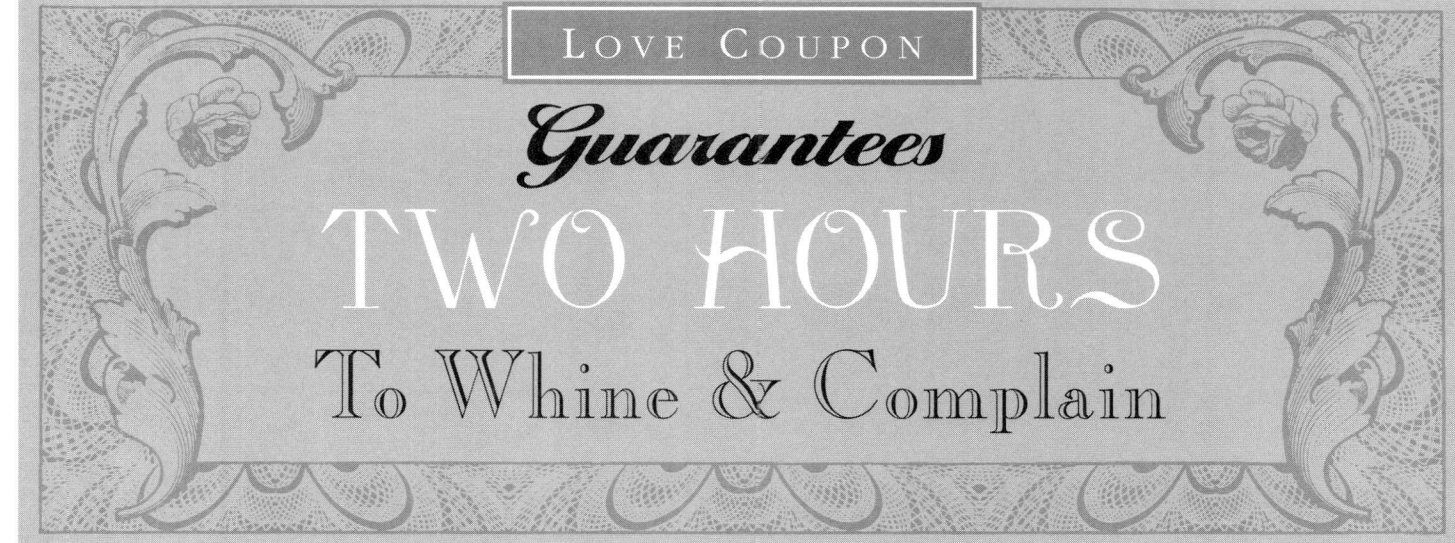

LOVE COUPON

Guarantees

TWO HOURS

To Whine & Complain

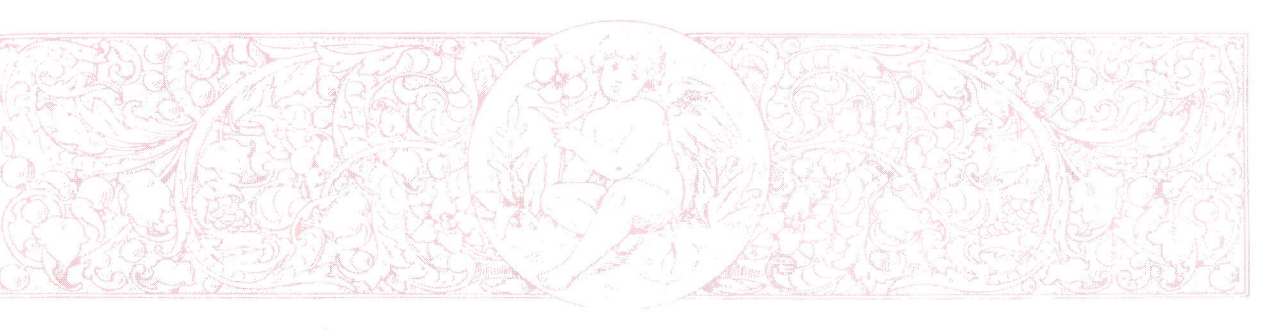

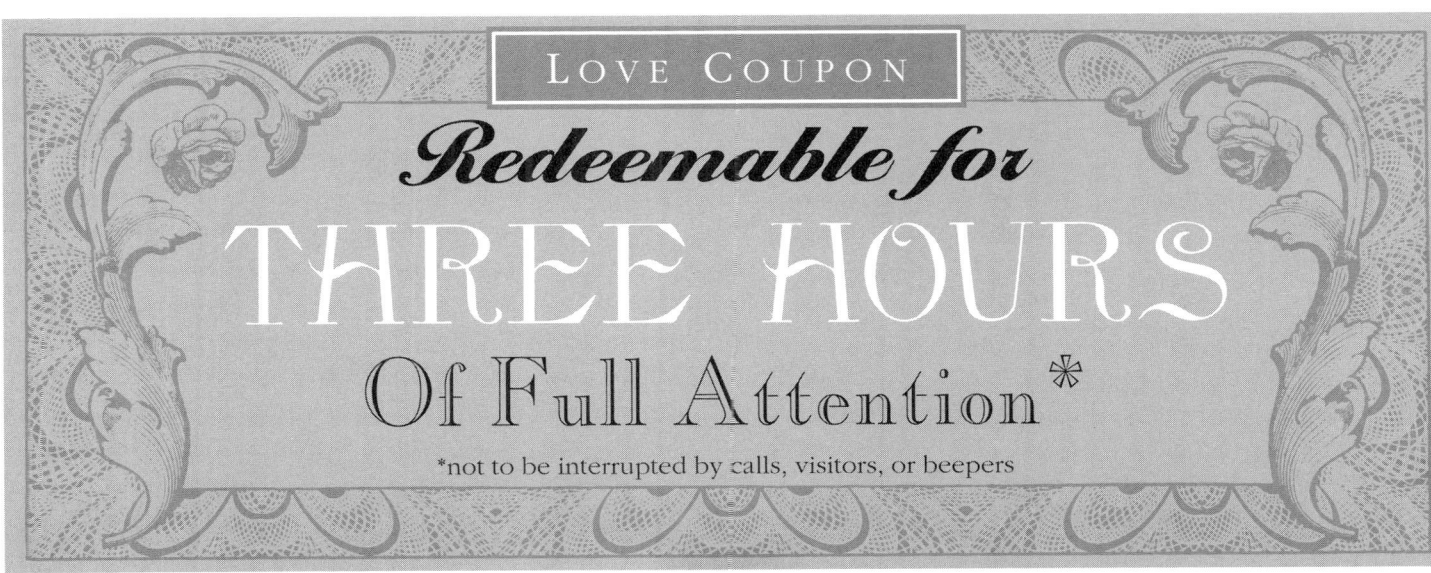

LOVE COUPON

Redeemable for

THREE HOURS

Of Full Attention*

*not to be interrupted by calls, visitors, or beepers

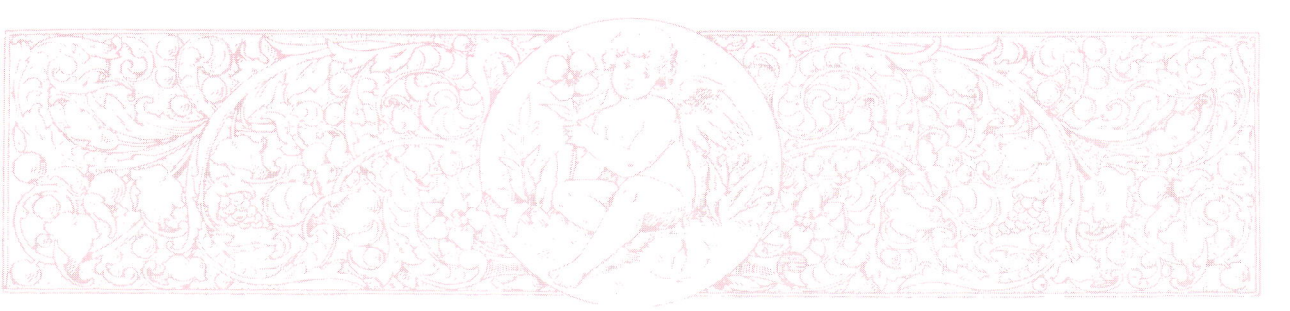

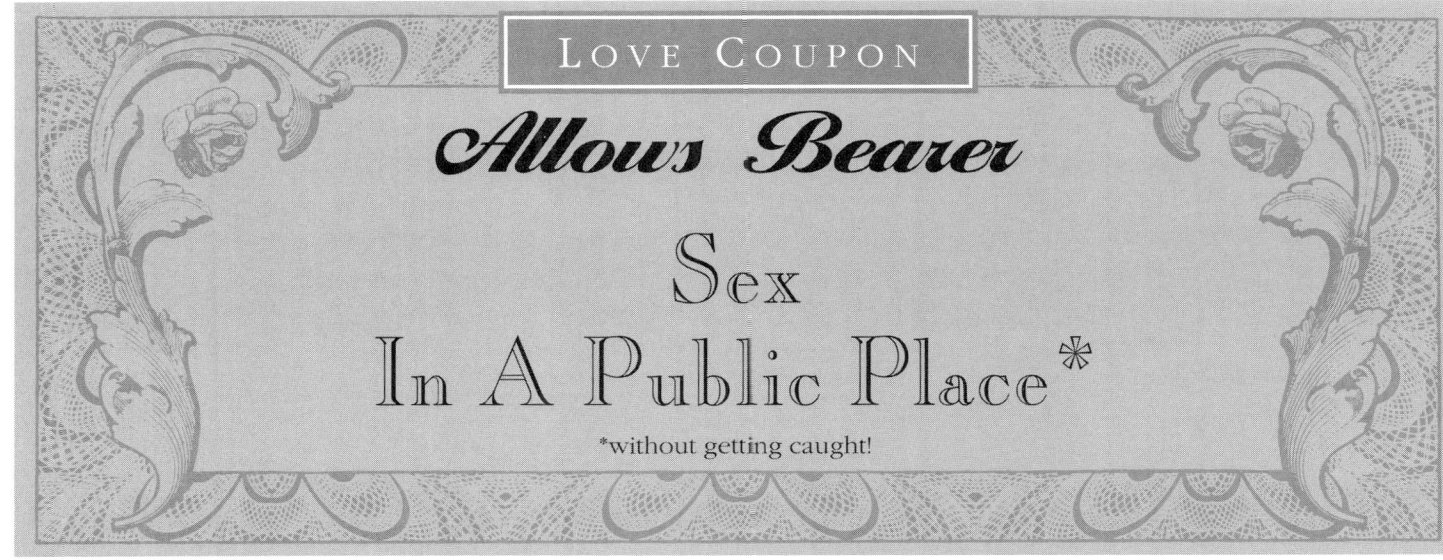

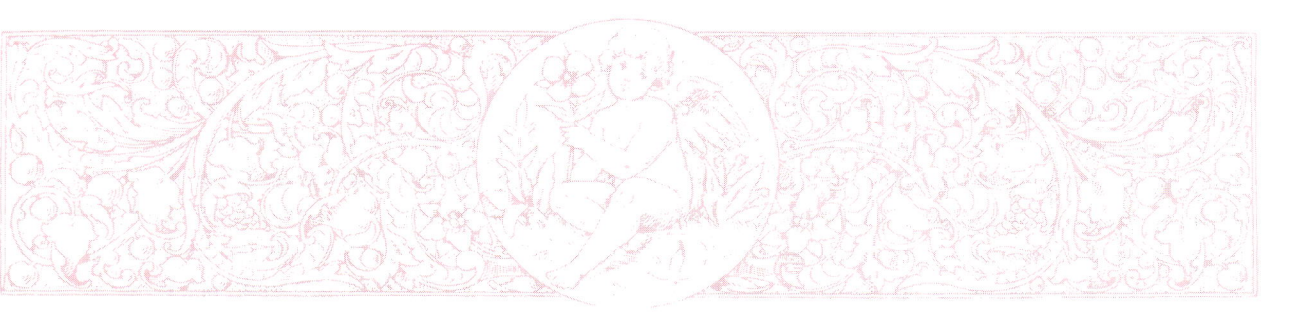

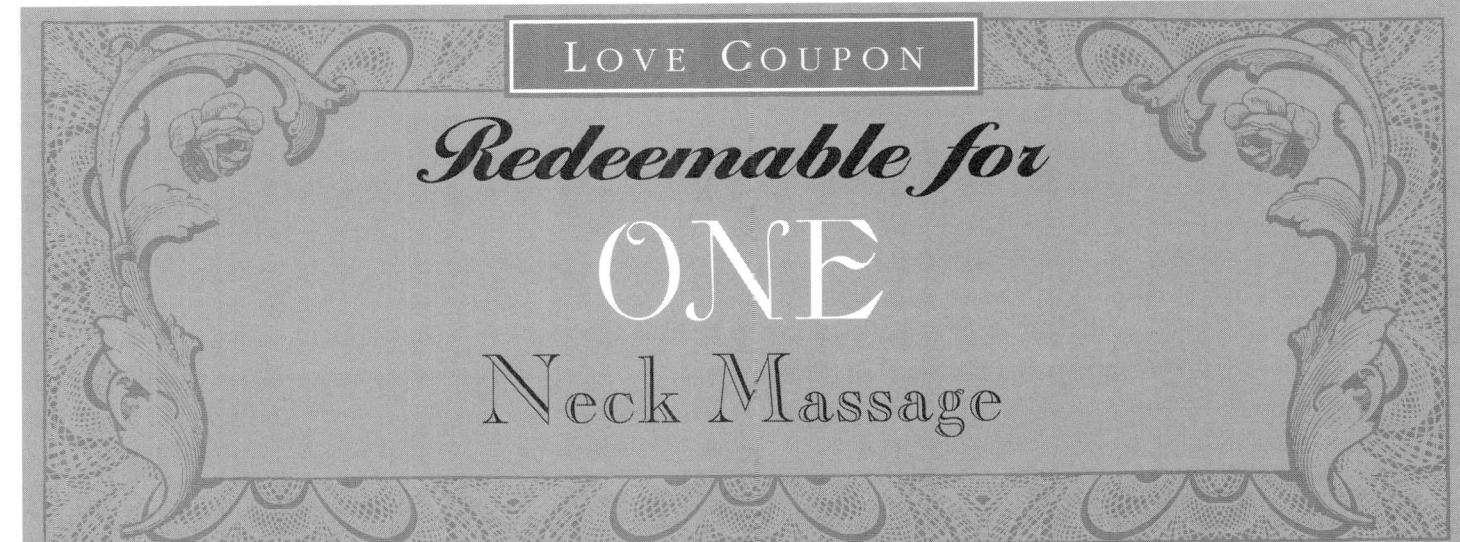

Love Coupon

Redeemable for

ONE

Neck Massage

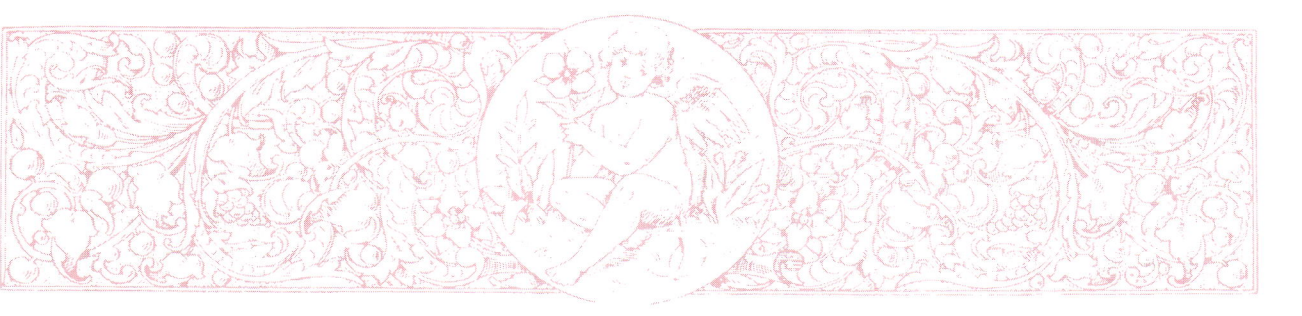

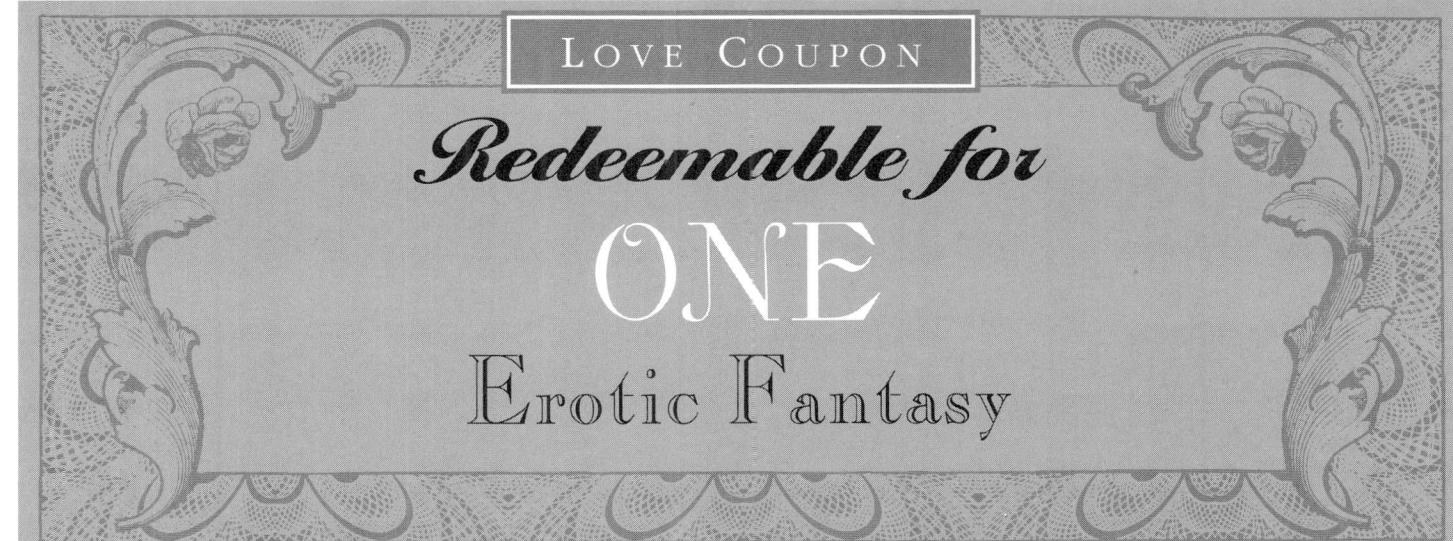

LOVE COUPON

Redeemable for

ONE

Erotic Fantasy

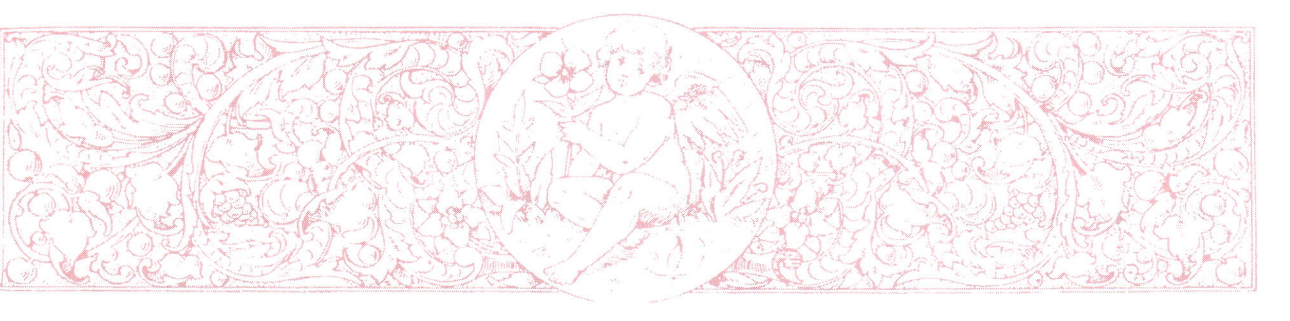

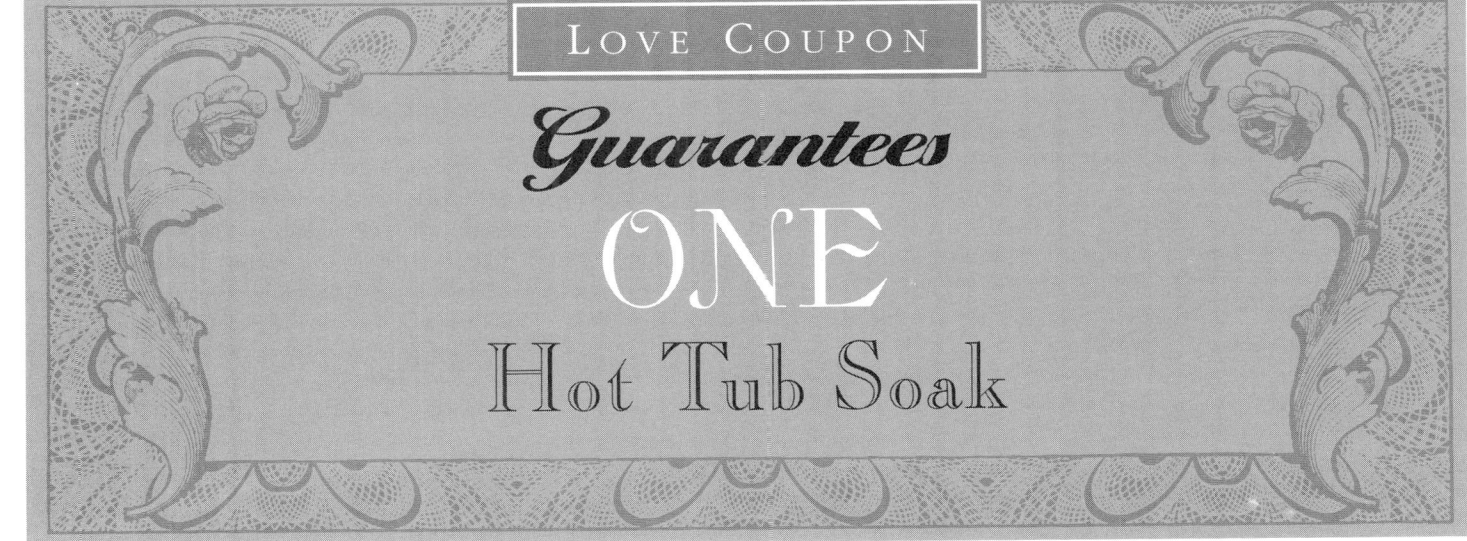

LOVE COUPON

Guarantees

ONE

Hot Tub Soak

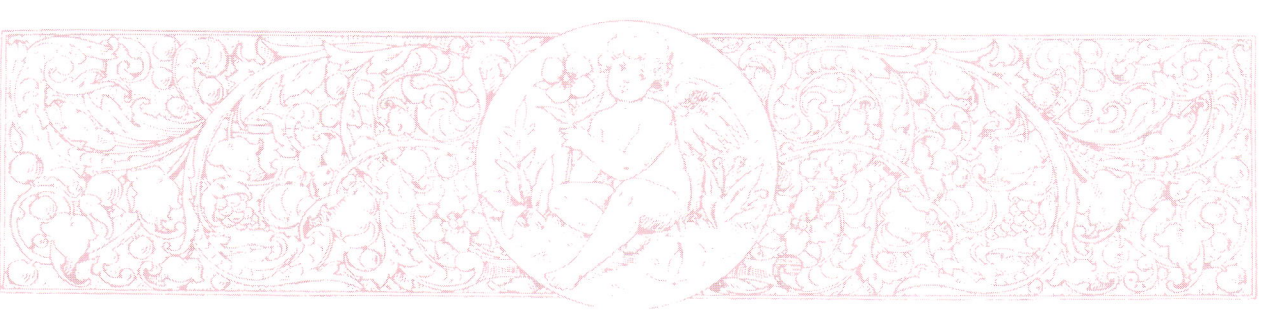

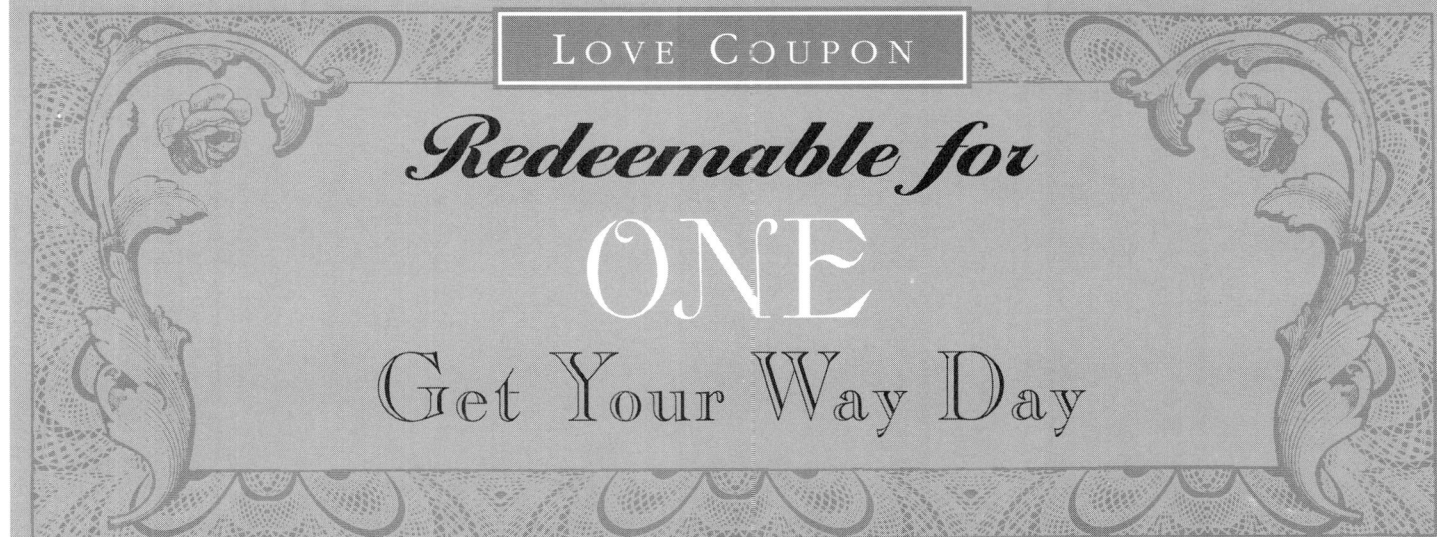

LOVE COUPON

Redeemable for

ONE

Get Your Way Day

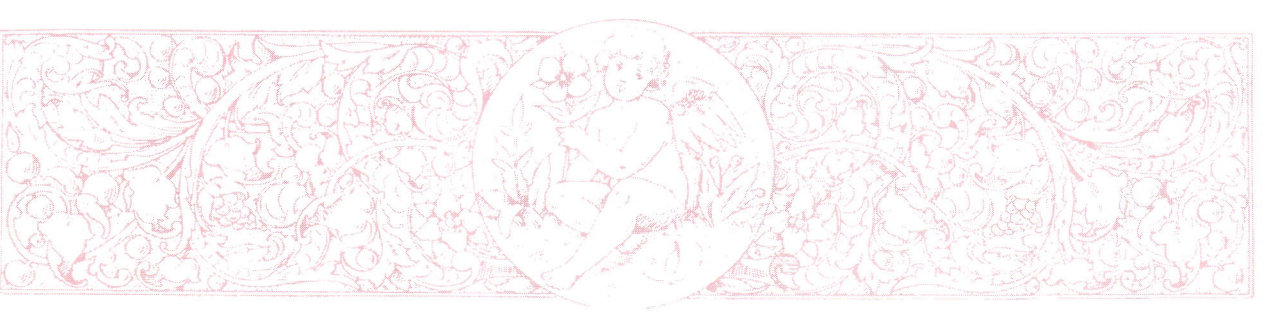

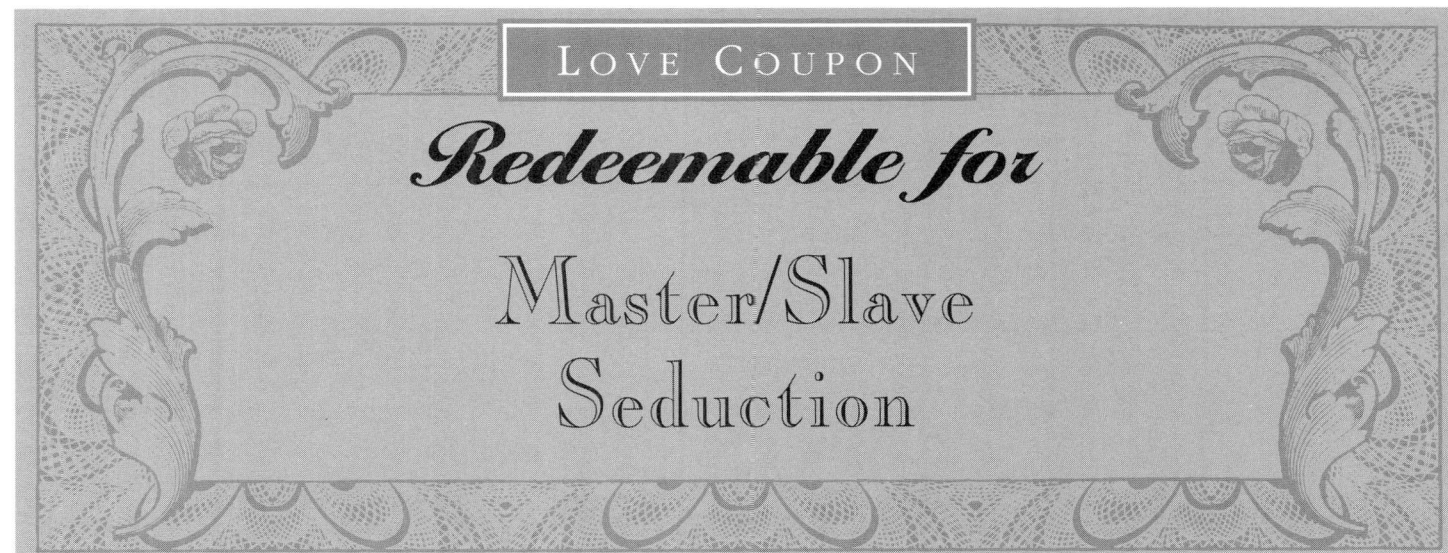

LOVE COUPON

Redeemable for

Master/Slave
Seduction

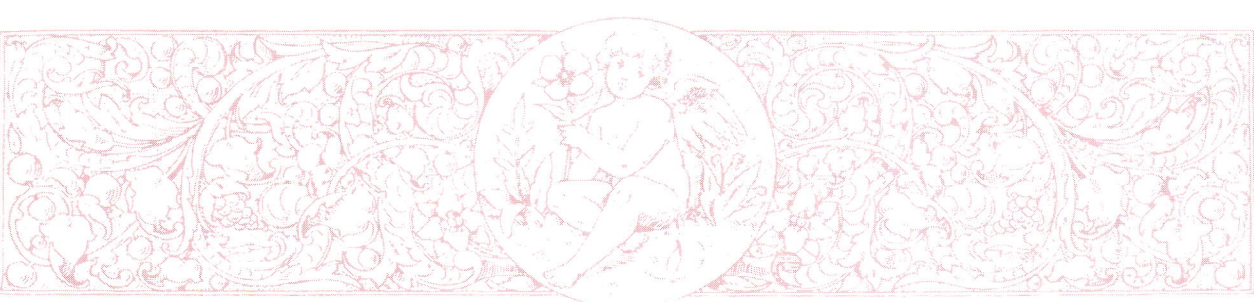

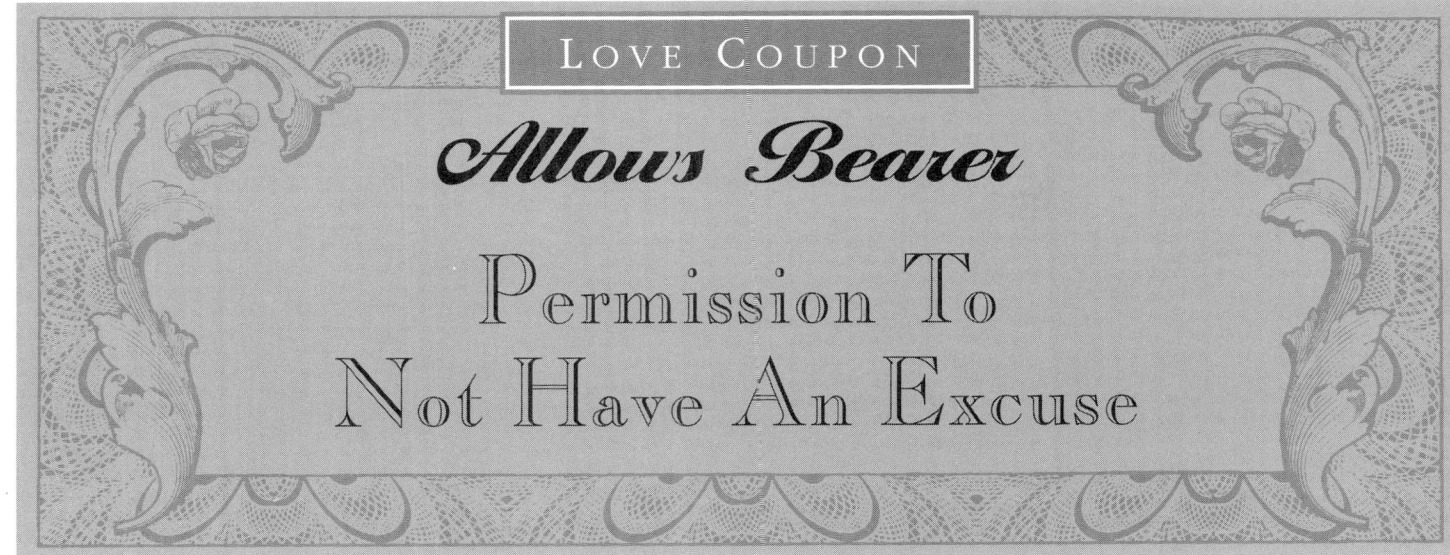

LOVE COUPON

Allows Bearer

Permission To
Not Have An Excuse

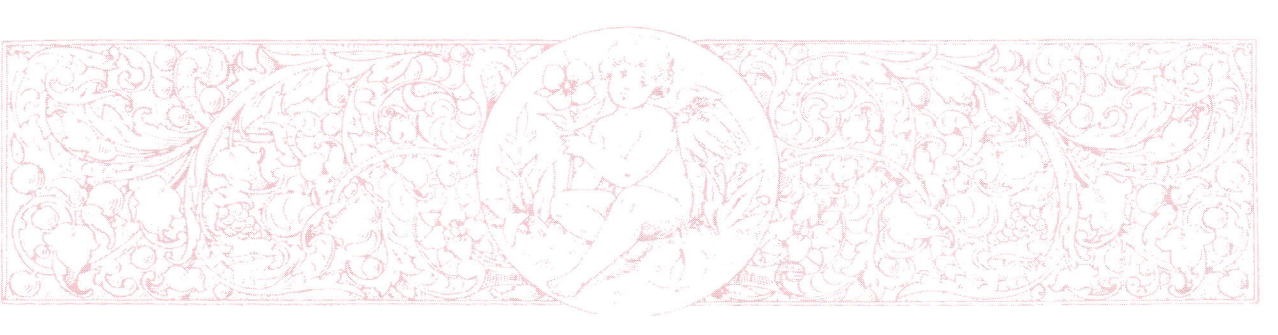

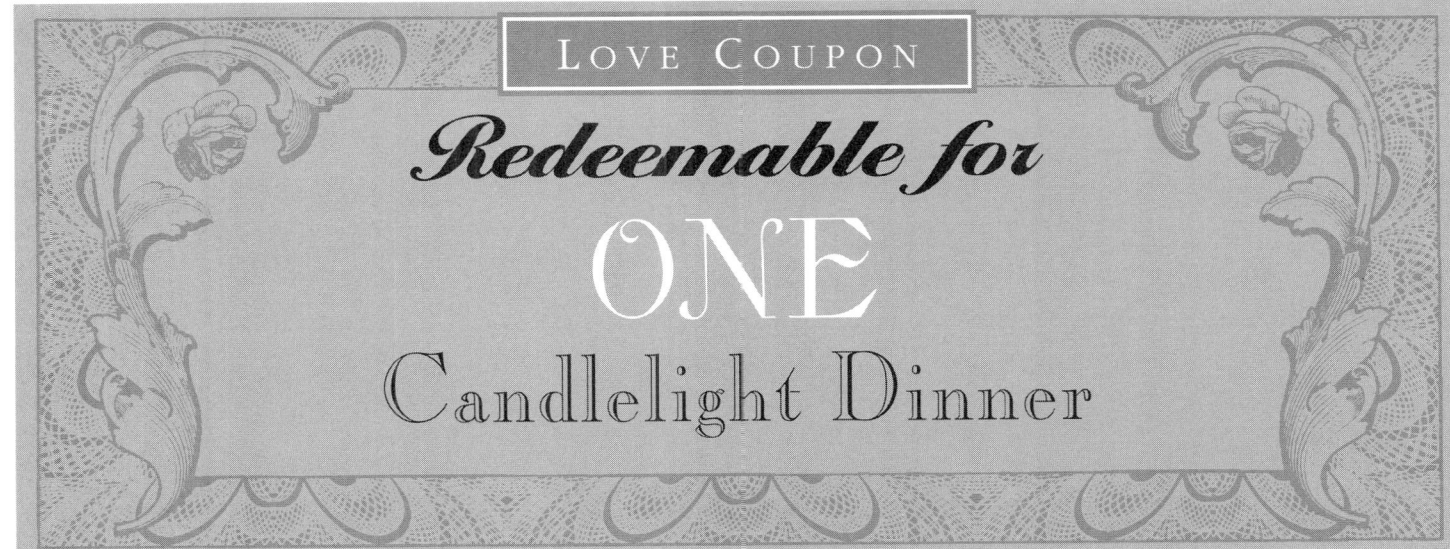

LOVE COUPON

Redeemable for

ONE

Candlelight Dinner

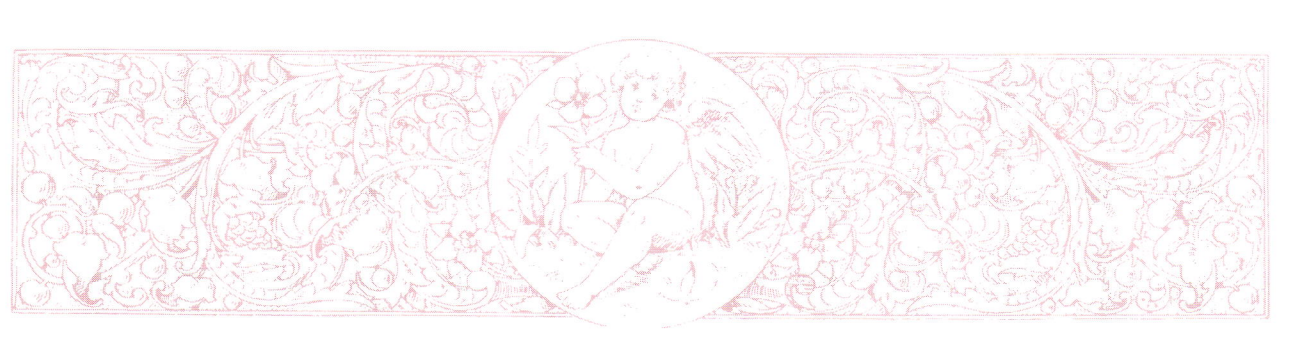

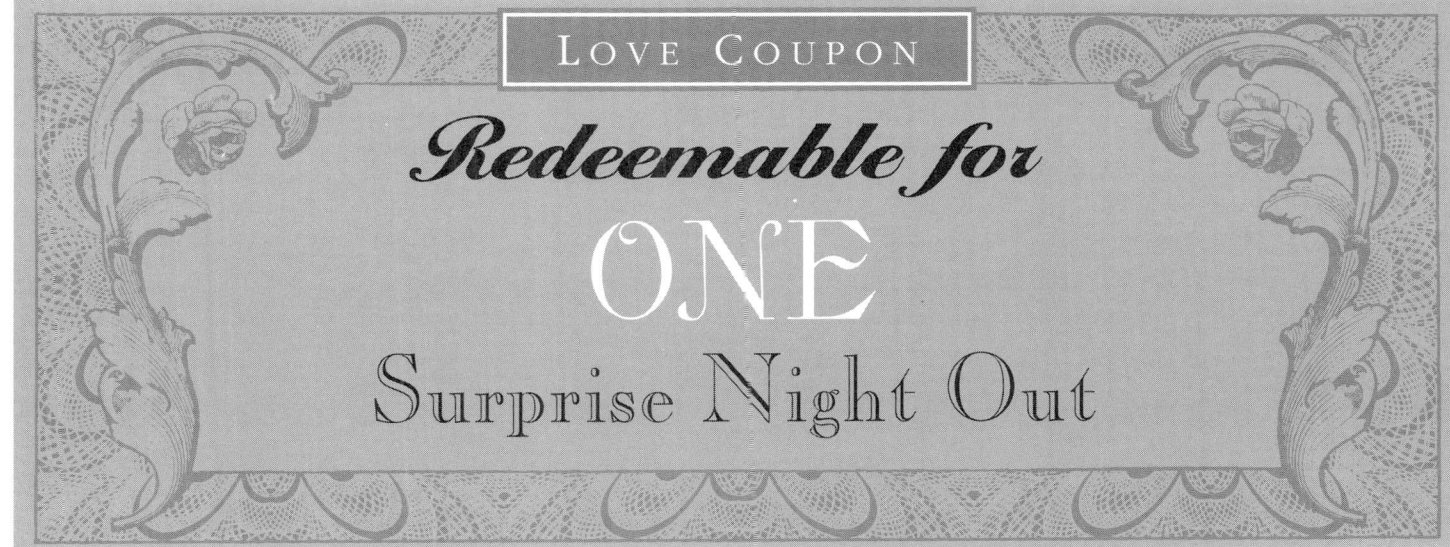

LOVE COUPON

Redeemable for

ONE

Surprise Night Out

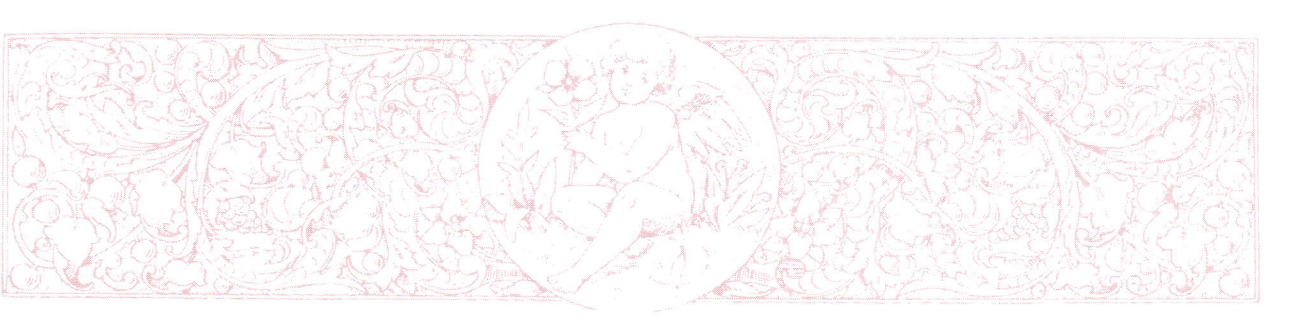

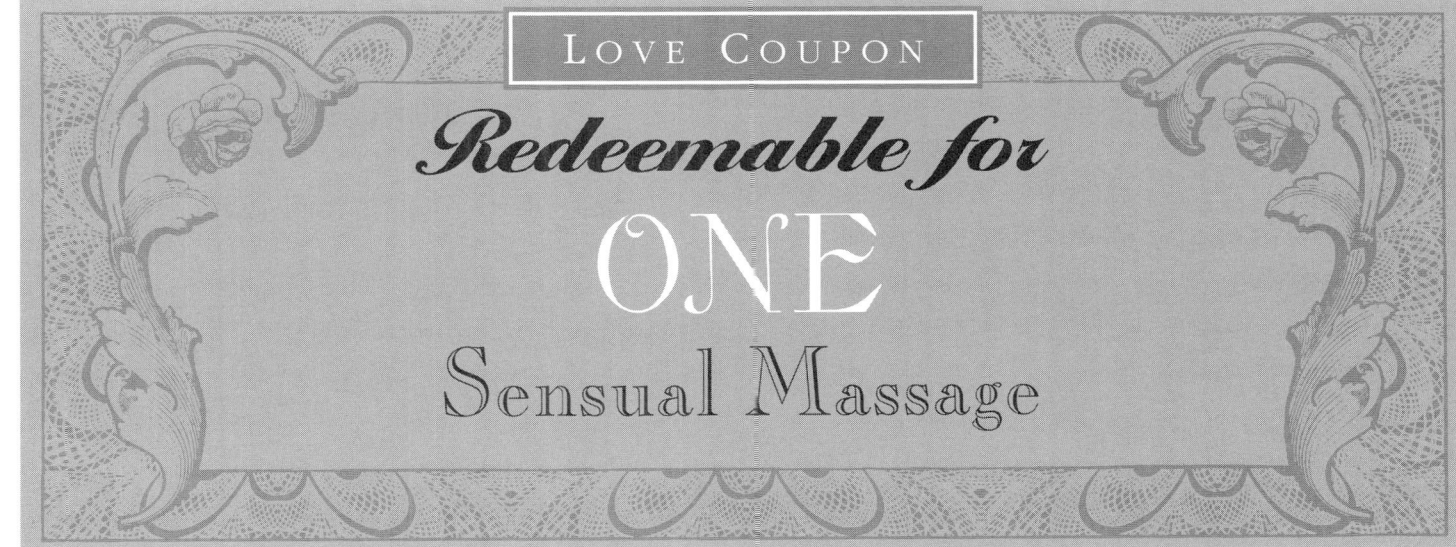

LOVE COUPON

Redeemable for

ONE

Sensual Massage

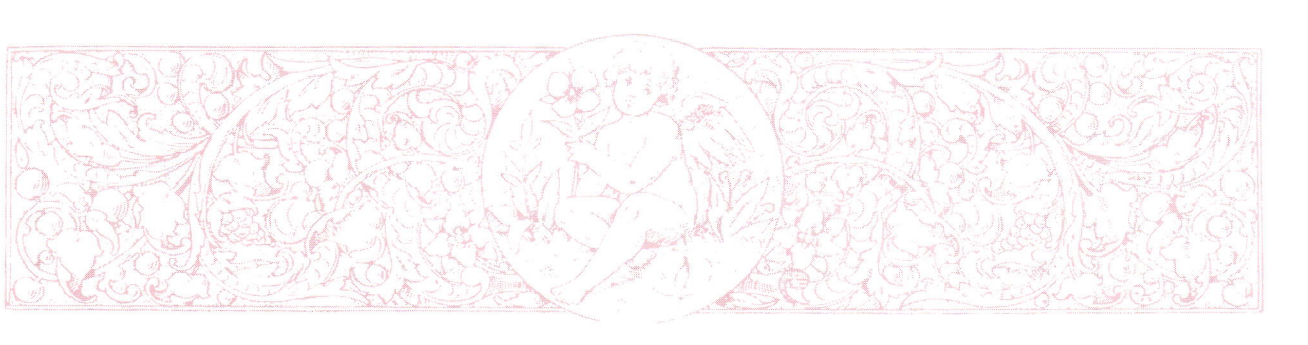

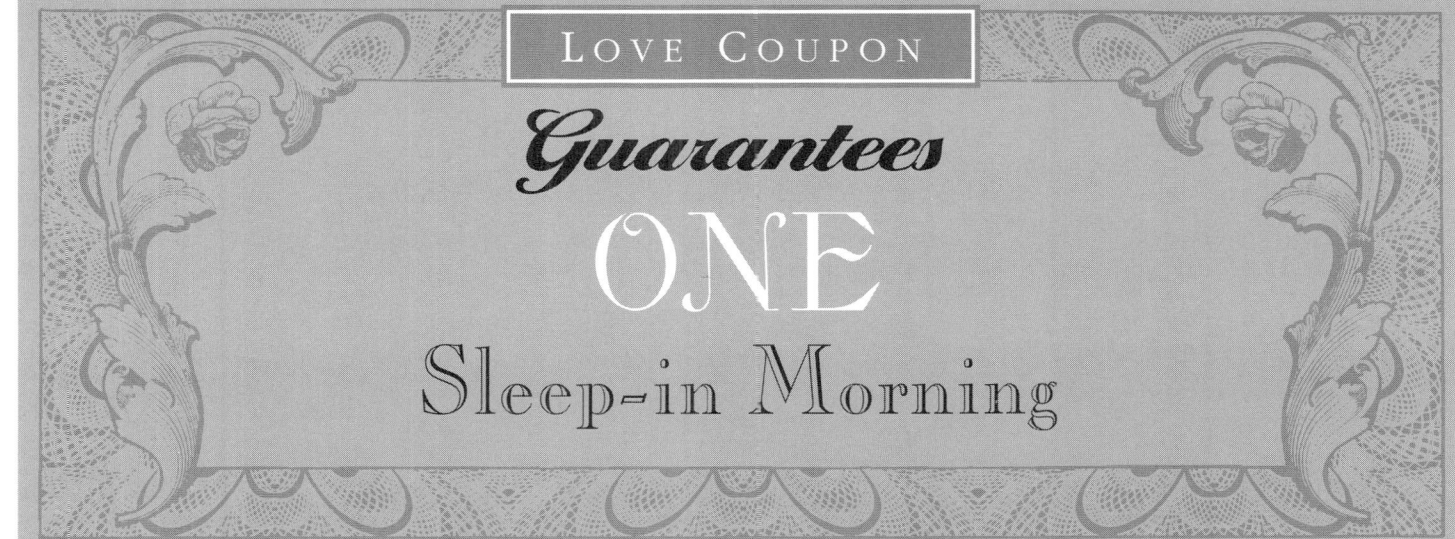

LOVE COUPON

Guarantees

ONE

Sleep-in Morning

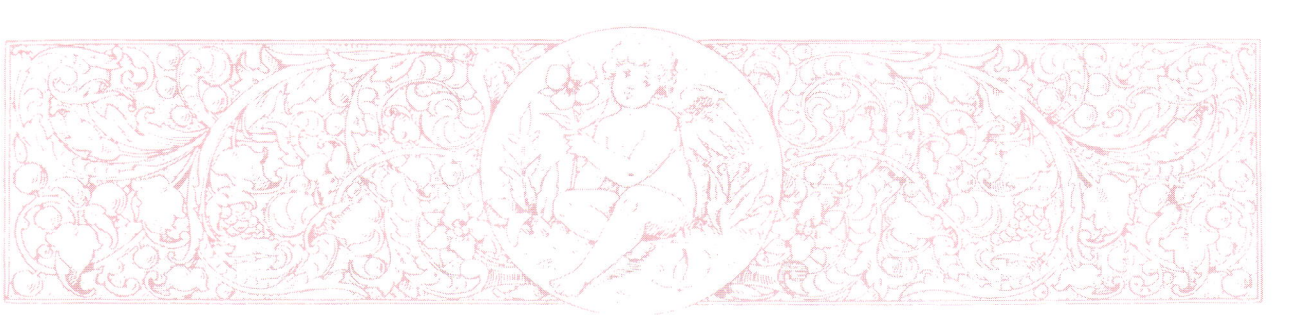

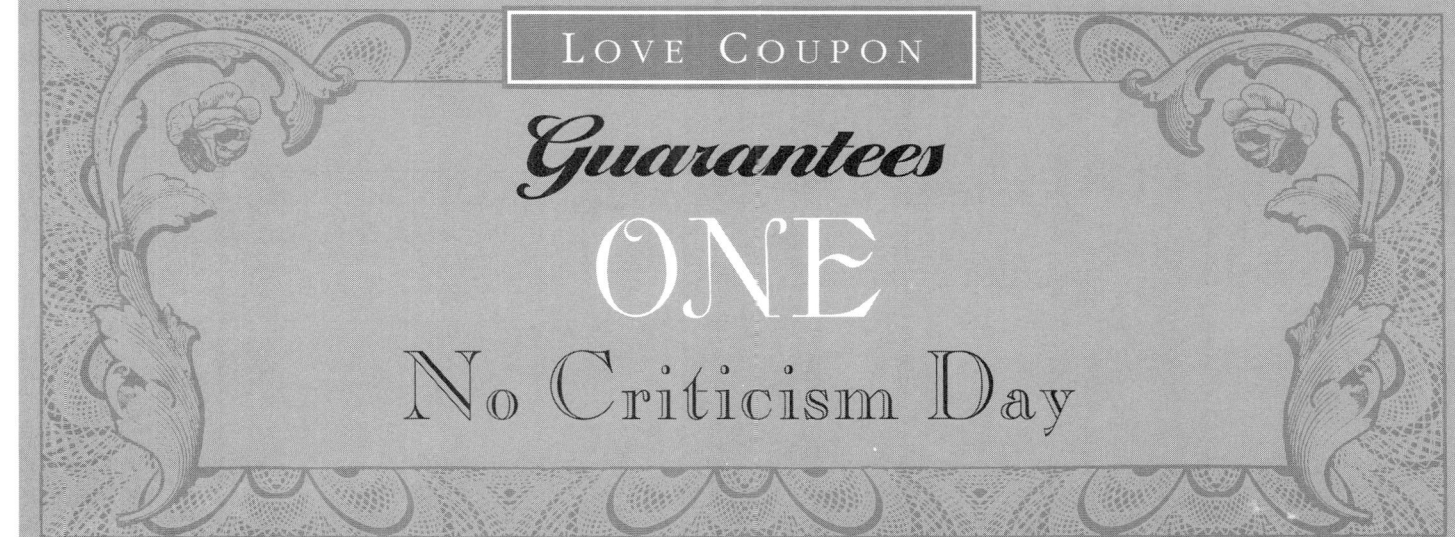

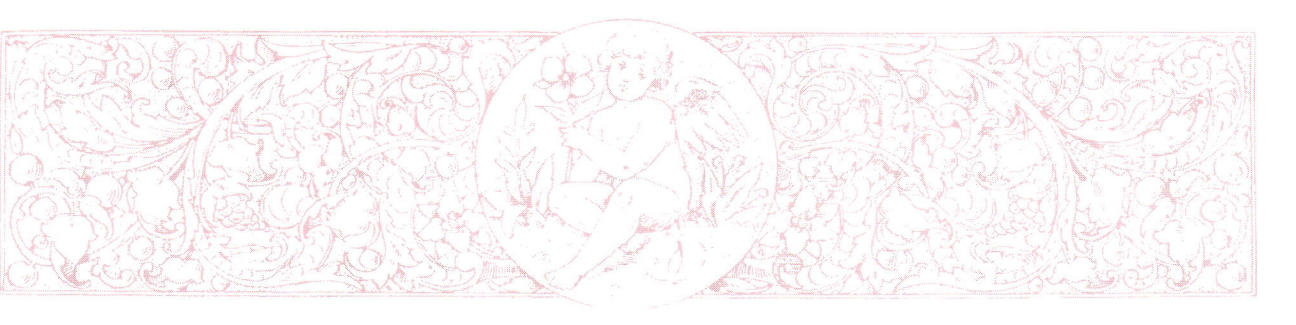

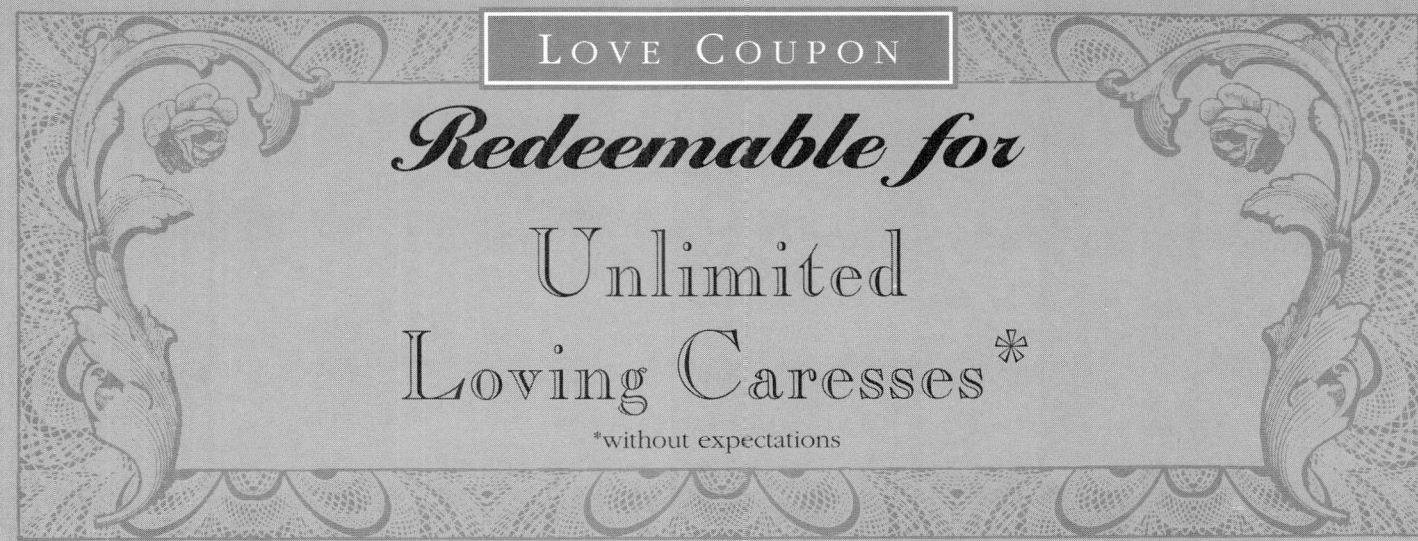

LOVE COUPON

Redeemable for

Unlimited
Loving Caresses*

*without expectations

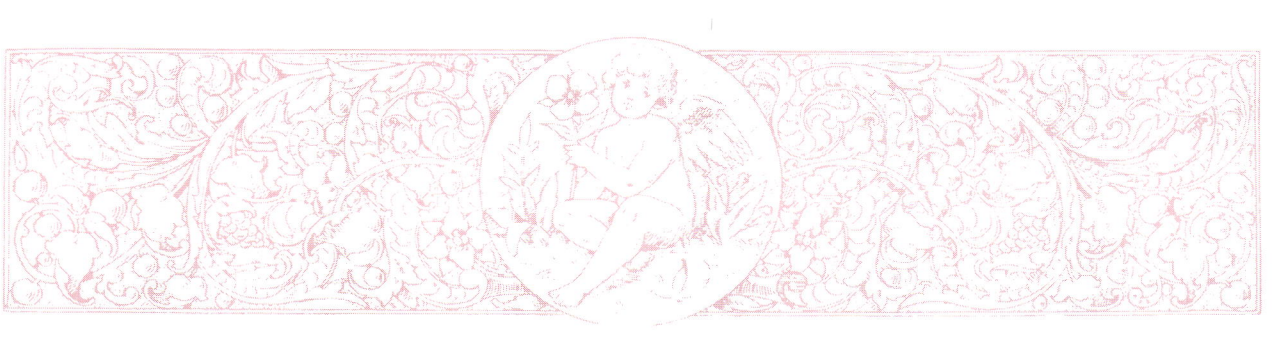

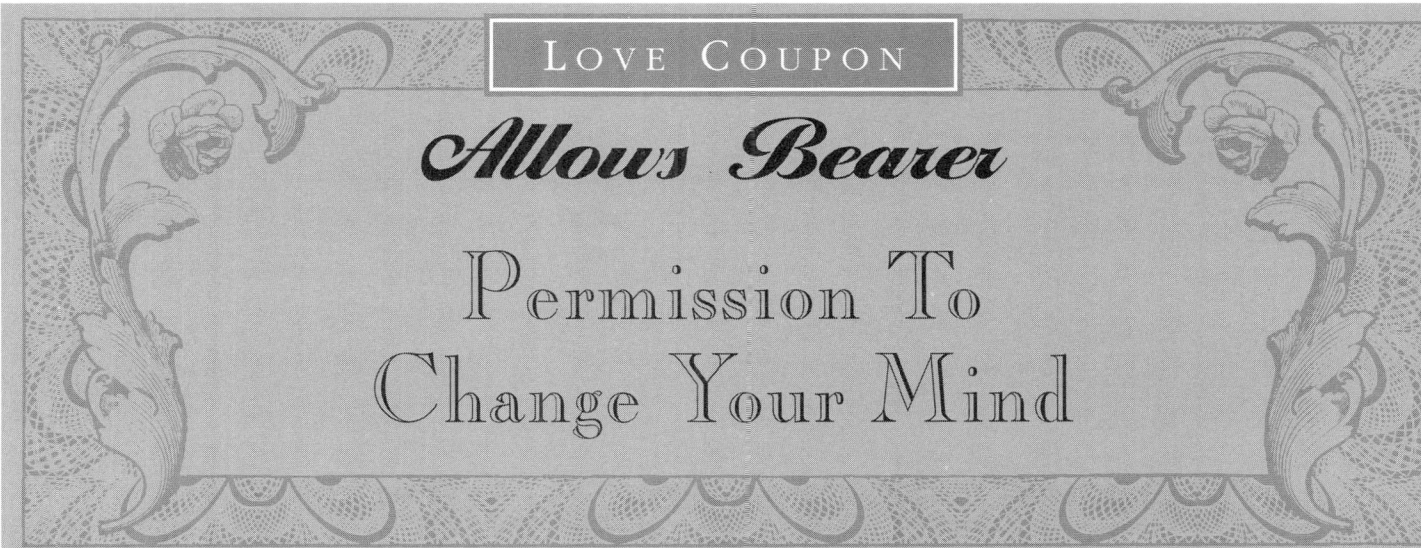

LOVE COUPON

Allows Bearer

Permission To
Change Your Mind

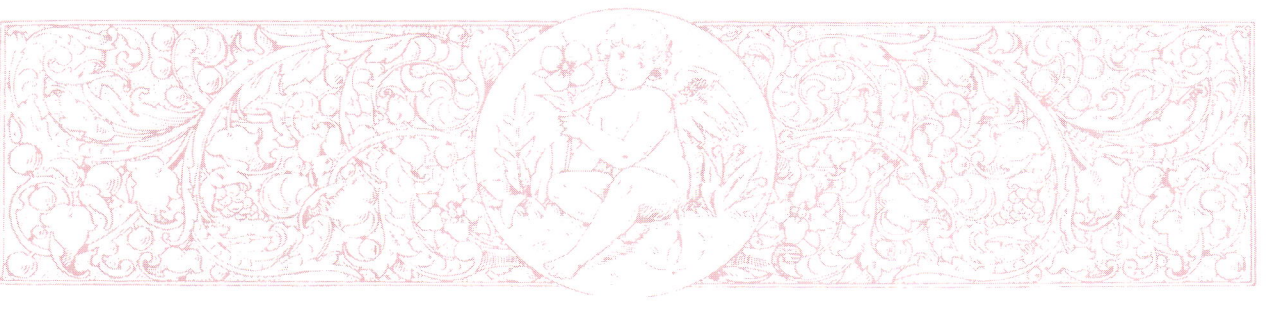

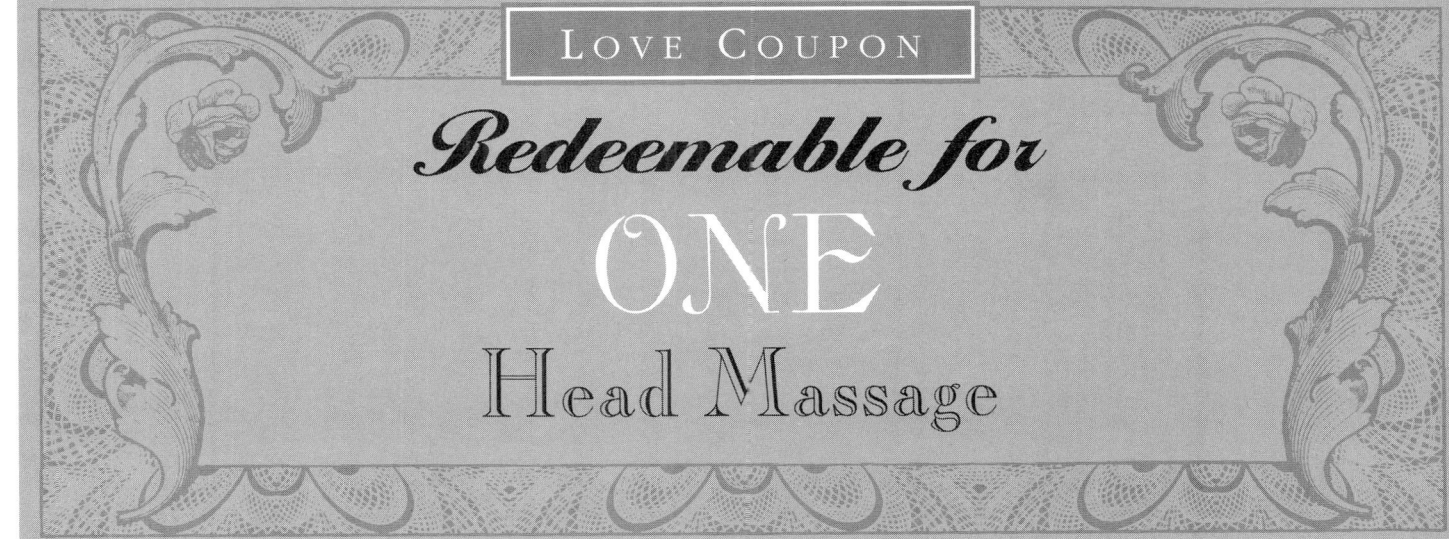

LOVE COUPON

Redeemable for

ONE

Head Massage

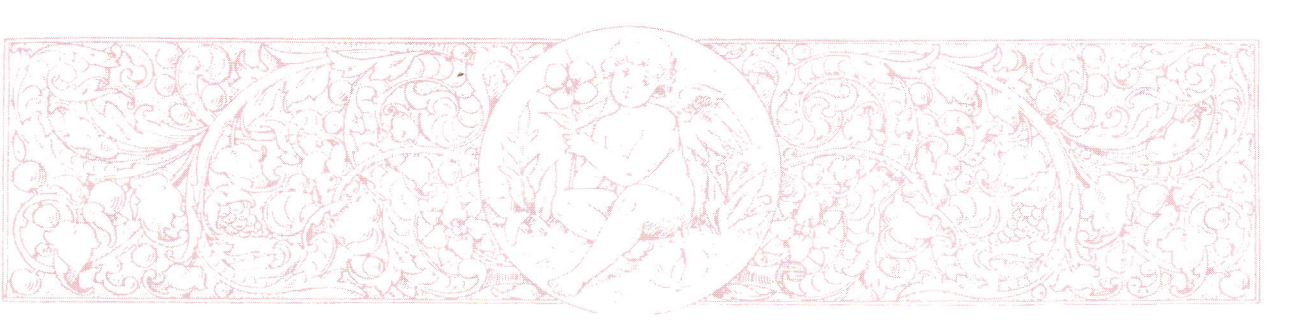

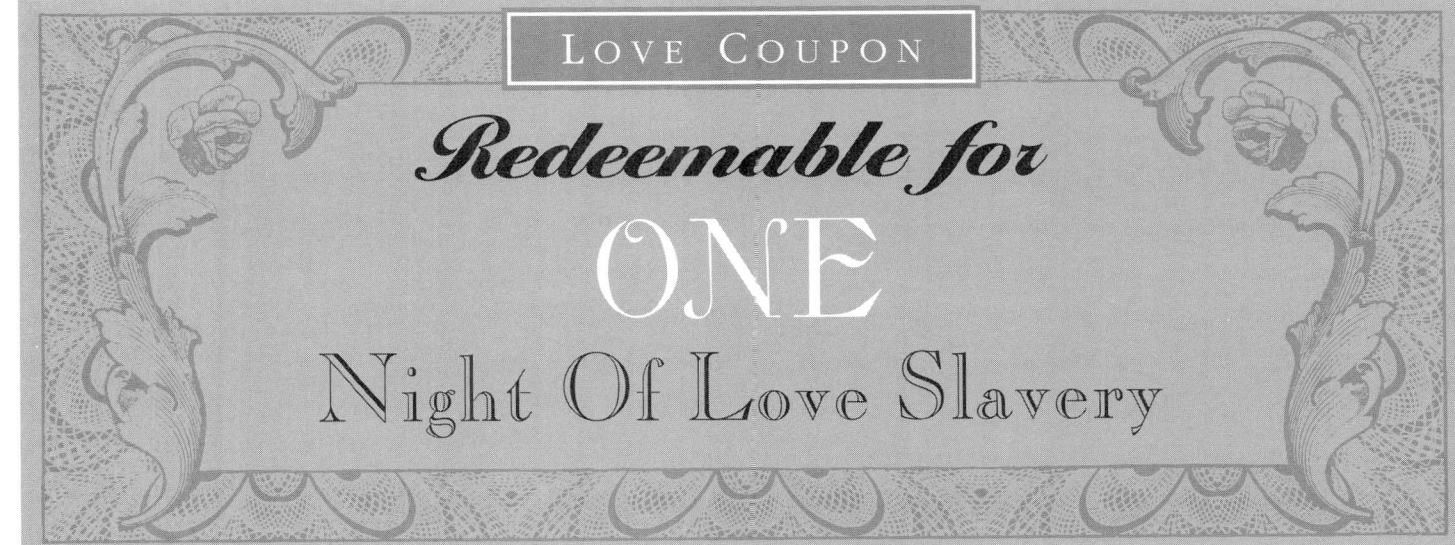

LOVE COUPON

Redeemable for

ONE

Night Of Love Slavery

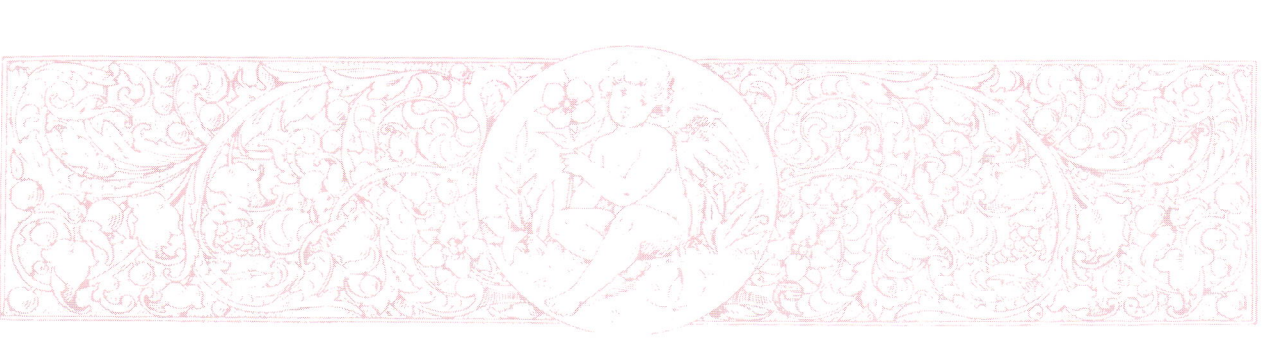

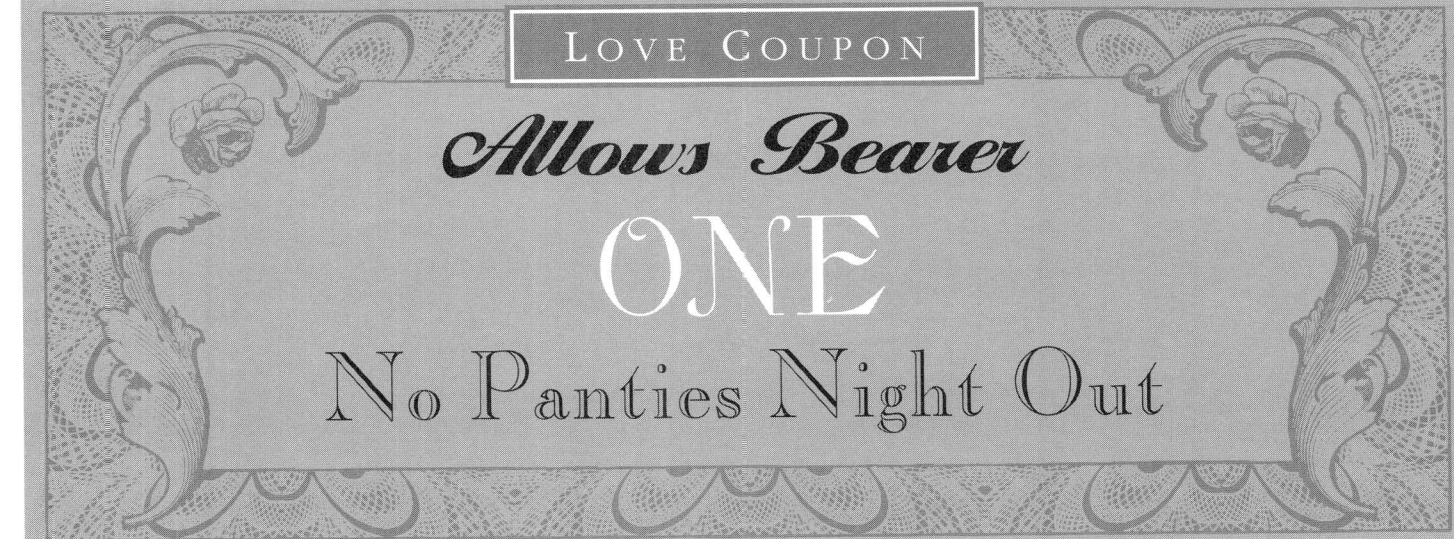

LOVE COUPON

Allows Bearer

ONE

No Panties Night Out

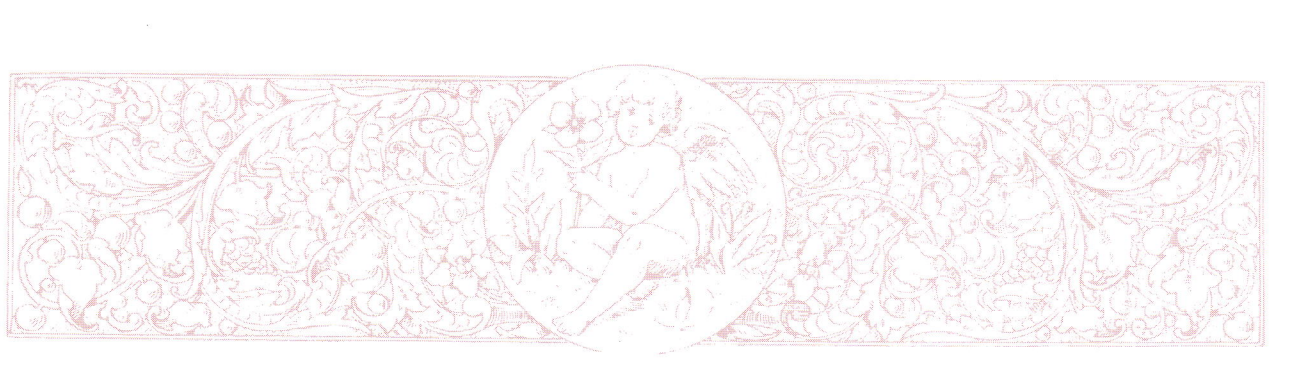

LOVE COUPON

Redeemable for

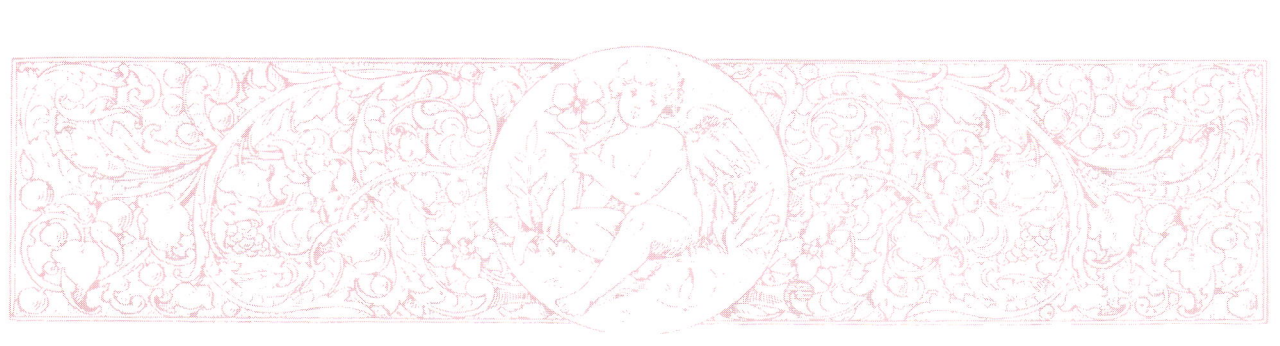

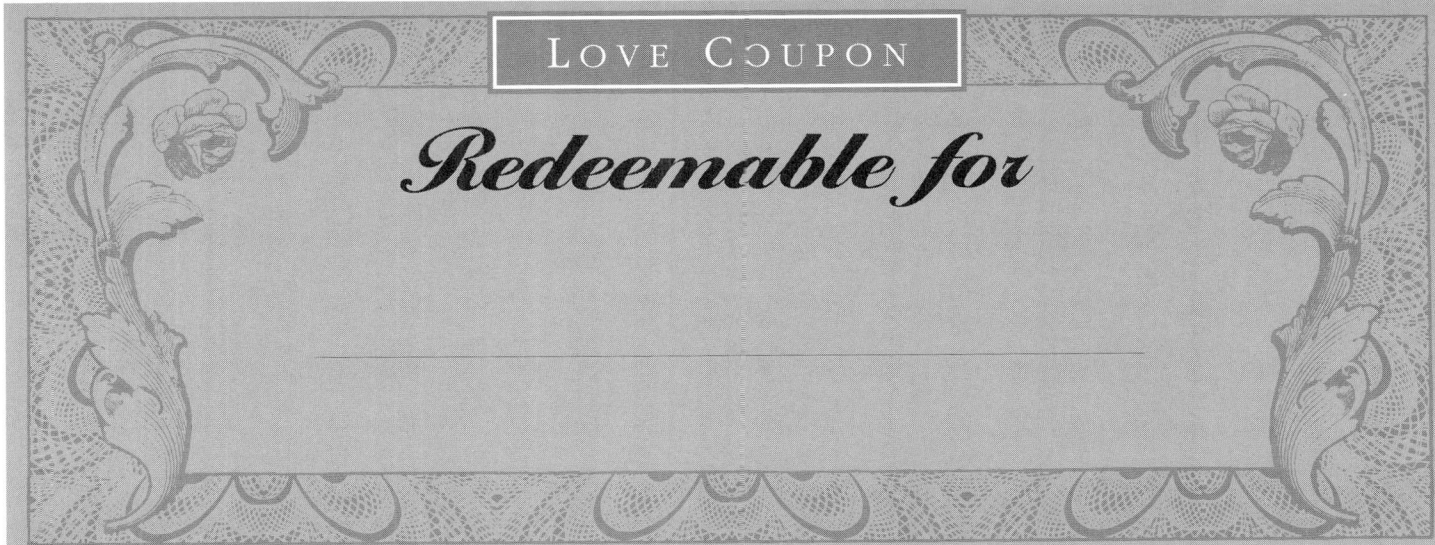

LOVE COUPON

Redeemable for

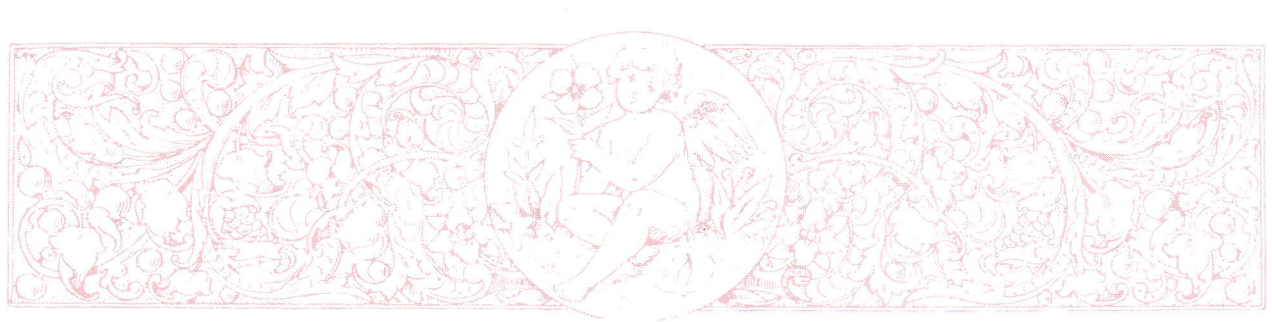